INFERTILITY MА̶

Practical Management of

MALE INFERTILITY

INFERTILITY MANAGEMENT SERIES

Practical Management of
MALE INFERTILITY

Series Editors

Juan A Garcia-Velasco MD PhD
Director-IVI Madrid, Spain
Associate Professor-Obstetrics and Gynecological
Madrid University, Spain

Manish Banker MD
Executive Director-Nova IVI Fertility, India
Director-Pulse Women's Hospital, Ahmedabad, India
Past President-Indian Society for Assisted Reproduction (ISAR)
Chairperson-Scientific Committee, IFFS 2016
Ahmedabad, India

Editor

Rupin Shah MS MCh (Urology)
Consultant Andrologist and Microsurgeon
Lilavati Hospital and Research Center, Mumbai, India
Consultant Andrologist-Nova IVI Fertility, India

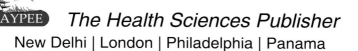

JAYPEE *The Health Sciences Publisher*
New Delhi | London | Philadelphia | Panama

Jaypee Brothers Medical Publishers (P) Ltd

Headquarters

Jaypee Brothers Medical Publishers (P) Ltd
4838/24, Ansari Road, Daryaganj
New Delhi 110 002, India
Phone: +91-11-43574357
Fax: +91-11-43574314
Email: jaypee@jaypeebrothers.com

Overseas Offices

J.P. Medical Ltd
83, Victoria Street, London
SW1H 0HW (UK)
Phone: +44-2031708910
Fax: +02-03-0086180
Email: info@jpmedpub.com

Jaypee-Highlights.
Medical Publishers Inc
City of Knowledge, Bld. 237
Clayton, Panama City, Panama
Phone: +1 507-301-0496
Fax: +1 507-301-0499
Email: cservice@jphmedical.com

Jaypee Medical Inc.
The Bourse
111 South Independence Mall East
Suite 835, Philadelphia
PA 19106, USA
Phone: +1 267-519-9789
Email: jpmed.us@gmail.com

Jaypee Brothers
Medical Publishers (P) Ltd
17/1-B Babar Road, Block-B
Shaymali, Mohammadpur
Dhaka-1207, Bangladesh
Mobile: +08801912003485
Email: jaypeedhaka@gmail.com

Jaypee Brothers
Medical Publishers (P) Ltd
Shorakhute, Kathmandu
Nepal
Phone: +00977-9841528578
Email: jaypee.nepal@gmail.com

Website: www.jaypeebrothers.com
Website: www.jaypeedigital.com

© 2015, Jaypee Brothers Medical Publishers

Inquiries for bulk sales may be solicited at: jaypee@jaypeebrothers.com

Infertility Management Series: Practical Management of Male Infertility

First Edition: 2015

ISBN 978-93-5152-570-7

Printed at: Samrat Offset Pvt. Ltd.

Dedicated to

The countless couples who have struggled, with patience and perseverance, through heartbreak and disappointment, to realize their dreams to bring new life to the world.

Contributors

Carlos Balmori MD FECMS
Consultant-Men's Health and Sexual Medicine, IVI-Madrid, Spain

Alberto Pacheco Castro PhD
Director-Andrology laboratory, IVI Madrid, Spain
Associate Professor-Alfonso X "El Sabio" University, Madrid, Spain

PM Gopinath MD DGO FMMC FICS FICOG MBA
Director-Institute of Ob Gyn and IVF, SRM Institutes for Medical Sciences
Vadapalani, Chennai, India

Vineet Malhotra MBBS, MS, DNB (Urology)
Consultant Urologist and Andrologist
Nova IVI Fertility, New Delhi, India
Rockland Hospital, New Delhi, India

Cristina González Ravina PhD
Director-Andrology laboratory, IVI Sevilla, Spain
Associate Professor-Seville University, Spain

Rupin Shah MS MCh (Urology)
Consultant Andrologist and Microsurgeon
Lilavati Hospital and Research Center, Mumbai, India
Consultant Andrologists-Nova IVI Fertility, India

Foreword

In this edition of the series of books reviewing the Human Reproduction we face the matter of the male factor. As in previous monographs the authors will try to offer a practical approach of this pathology.

Male factor has been frequently considered to be a minor issue as opposed to female factor considering the strong relevance of the oocyte although this is a mistaken approach if we understand that male pathology is responsible for a high percentage of cases of sterility. If we carry out a correct diagnosis of the male and his semen sample we will be able to find the best way to tackle this pathology and, therefore, improve the condition of the couple when facing their sterility problem.

Over the years we are witnessing an enthralling emergence of new approaches for the diagnosis of the male factor including its genetic study.

I hope this handbook can be very useful in your daily practice and I encourage Nova IVI Fertility to go on with this way of continuous training for professionals working in the exciting area of human reproduction.

Antonio Requena
Director, Medico General Equipo IVI
Director, IVI Madrid, Spain

Preface

The male has long been ignored in the evaluation of an infertile couple.

In the past, it was because the male himself was usually reluctant to come for evaluation, and the burden of infertility fell upon the woman. Later, even when semen analysis became common, evaluation and management of the male remained secondary due to the lack of therapeutic options. Then, when ICSI became the ultimate answer to male subfertility, ironically it shifted the spotlight away from the male because the infertility specialist used whatever sperm were available without being concerned about how to improve their number or quality.

However, recently the focus has finally shifted to the male due to the realization that merely having sperm is not enough, and that subnormal sperm will compromise pregnancy outcomes after ICSI. Hence, men are now being assessed thoroughly to assess their fertility potential, and are being treated when this is found to be suboptimal. Further, an increasing number of genetic causes of male infertility are being identified, with clinical and therapeutic implications and finally, advances in microsurgical techniques for reconstruction in obstructive azoospermia and for retrieving sperm in non-obstructive azoospermia have brought new hope to previously hopelessly infertile couples, making it imperative that men with azoospermia be evaluated and managed correctly.

This practical handbook seeks to update the clinician with clinically relevant advances in this field. The first two chapters discuss the new WHO guidelines for semen analysis and the use of special tests to assess sperm function, especially DNA integrity. Subsequent chapters address the uncommon but frustrating practical problem of ejaculatory failure, the treatment of OATS through medical and surgical therapy, and the clinical approach to the evaluation and management for azoospermia—a subject of increasing importance.

It is hoped that this handbook will serve as a handy update and reference volume to the gynecologist dealing with infertile couples.

Rupin Shah

Contents

CHAPTER
1

Understanding the New WHO Semen Parameters

Cristina González Ravina, Alberto Pacheco Castro

INTRODUCTION

As it is well known, the first *Laboratory Manual for the Analysis of Human Semen and Its Interaction with the Cervical Mucus* was published in 1980. This was as a response to the high necessity of standardizing the protocols to carry out this analysis.[1] This manual has subsequently been reviewed three times. In 2010, the 5th edition of the *Laboratory Manual for the Examination and Processing of Human Semen* was published. In this edition, the latest so far, the reference values, the algorithms for diagnosis, the clinical interpretation of diagnosis, and other relevant aspects have been reviewed. Until last year, every andrology or assisted reproduction laboratory worked according to the guidelines recommended in the latest manuals published by the WHO.[1-3]

After making a revision of these manuals and the reference values that existed up to the year 2010, it can be observed that they were useful when established in 1999, but nowadays an update of these was necessary. It should be remembered that the studies performed to establish the reference values in 1999 were based in the analysis of two semen samples from a not-very-high number of males in different laboratories where the work method had not yet been standardized nor the pertinent quality systems had yet been introduced.

THE PREVIOUS WHO MANUAL

In the manual published in 1999, spermatozoa were classified in four categories regarding their motility: type a [rapid progressive motility (PM)], type b (slow PM), type c [nonprogressive motility (NP)], and type d [immotility (IM)]. One of the main restrictions from this classification is the acknowledgement that sperm PM (types a + b) studies and morphology studies

Table 1.1: The reference values established in the WHO Laboratory Manual of 1999.	
Seminal parameter	*Lower reference value*
• Volume	2.0 mL
• pH	7.2
• Concentration	20 million spermatozoa per milliliter
• Total number of spermatozoa	40 million spermatozoa per ejaculation
• Motility	50% type a + b spermatozoa per ejaculation 25% type a spermatozoa per ejaculation
• Vitality	75% spermatozoa alive per ejaculation
• Morphology	15% normal shape

were not only subjective but also they did not follow any standard protocol in the laboratories.[4–6] However, the values obtained regarding sperm concentration and total motility (a + b + c) were considered acceptable. This is because they could be measured in a reproducible way in most centers. For this reason, it was recommended that each laboratory established their own limit values of normality for these variables, and they were also advised to include the appropriate internal and external quality assurances. These quality assurances are fully developed in the new manual of 2010.

In spite of this, reference ranges for the main seminal parameters were defined through a statistics analysis by comparing the sperm characteristics of a group of males. These reference ranges distinguished two different populations studied (fertile vs subfertile or subfertile vs infertile).[7,8]

The reference values established in 1999 are shown in Table 1.1.

Regarding morphology, the WHO Manual discusses the start of a multicenter study for the analysis of seminal parameters. The edition of 1999 specifies that the data obtained in centers with assisted reproduction programs suggest a connection between morphology values < 15% and a decrease in IVF (in vitro fertilization) rate.[9]

Regarding the nomenclature, these are the terms used to express seminogram values lower than the reference values:

- *Asthenozoospermia*: PM < 50% types a + b or < 25% type a
- *Oligozoospermia*: Concentration < 20 million/mL
- *Teratozoospermia*: Morphology < 15% normal shapes
- *Necrozoospermia*: Vitality < 75%
- *Cryptozoospermia*: Absence of spermatozoa in the first analysis of the ejaculation sample and presence of spermatozoa after centrifugation
- *Azoospermia*: Absence of spermatozoa in the first analysis of the ejaculation sample and absence of spermatozoa after centrifugation; concentration = 0
- *Aspermia*: Absence of ejaculation; volume = 0

Based on the male's seminal classification, his medical history and his physical exploration, as well as any other additional information, a diagnosis of the male could be given through a diagram based on different sperm concentration ranging from azoospermia, cryptozoospermia, and oligozoospermia samples.[1–3] It should be emphasized that in the manual of 1999 a subclassification for the different seminal alterations (oligo-, asteno-, terato-, necrozoospermia) is used, with a range from mild to moderate to severe.

CHANGES IN THE NEW 2010 WHO MANUAL

Eleven years after the edition of 1999, a review and update of the reference values and the established work protocols became more and more necessary. Therefore, the new online edition of the WHO manual of 2010 presents much more detail regarding seminal analysis: work solutions, procedures, calculations, and results interpretation. Furthermore, it recommends using a specific method in those cases in which there is more than one possible analysis technique.

Considering this, the main changes in the fifth edition include the following:

- A new work protocol to determine sperm concentration. The recommended semen dilutions and the counting chamber areas necessary to establish the number of spermatozoa (concentration) in order to count 200 spermatozoa by replicate have been modified. The goal of reducing sampling errors has been intensified, giving more importance to the sample volume, which was not so relevant before. This sample volume must be measured with precision and using the method recommended by the WHO manual.
- Regarding azoospermia, there is a change in the work protocols to be followed on this type of samples, in which there are no spermatozoa in the ejaculate. It differentiates the necessity to obtain a concentration value and/or an accurate motility value from centrifuging the sample to increase the chances of finding spermatozoa after washing.
- There are significant changes in the sperm motility classification. From now on, spermatozoa should be only differentiated according to three categories: PM—combining former types a + b, NP—former type c, and IM—former type d.
- The morphology analysis is dealt with in more detail in this edition. It includes pictures of spermatozoa considered normal and spermatozoa with one or several morphological anomalies, as well as accurate explanations to improve the technician's training regarding the study of this seminal parameter.
- On the other hand, the manual includes an improved chapter on semen cryopreservation, with a well-described section on sperm preparation.

It also dedicates a full chapter to quality assurance that, apart from being the novelty, involves a recommendation from the WHO to have quality assurance in our laboratories. This includes both the external and the internal quality assurance.

Therefore, the fifth edition of the Manual is divided into three parts:

- Semen analysis (Chapters 2–4)
  1. Standard procedures
  2. Optional procedures
  3. Research procedures
- Sperm preparation (Chapters 5 and 6)
- Quality assurance (Chapter 7)

METHODOLOGY AND INCLUSION CRITERIA

For this study, semen samples from 4,500 males from 14 countries and four continents were analyzed. They were divided into three wide groups: fertile males, males with unknown fertility, and normozoospermic males according to the manual of 1999. The group of males whose partner had become pregnant in a time period ≤12 months was selected as the control group to establish the reference values of seminal parameters (1,953 males, five studies in eight countries from three continents).

All the laboratories participating in this study obtained their data by using the standard methods of semen analysis.[1-2] Each laboratory was taken into account at the moment of assessing the results because this manual offers different methods to determine volume, sperm concentration, and morphological stain. Moreover, many laboratories implemented with delay the internal and external quality assurances. For this reason, the data were reviewed to calculate the reference distribution considering that fact.[10]

For this study, only one ejaculated semen sample per male, which was gathered with a sexual abstinence period of 2–7 days, was used. Concentration was measured in most cases with the improved Neubauer hemocytometer. Motility data were gathered on total motility (WHO 1999: a + b + c) and PM (WHO 1999: a + b).[11] Morphology data were taken into account only in those centers using Tygerberg's strict criteria.[1-3] Finally, vitality, analyzed by eosin-nigrosin staining, got a significantly lower number of samples studied than the other seminal parameters, only two centers provided data. The advantage of having standard work protocols is that the analytic error has been minimized and the values presented are considered representative of the seminal characteristics of a fertile male.

NEW REFERENCE VALUES AND DIAGNOSIS

This edition reviews old reference values and establishes new ones with which we have to work nowadays (Table 1.2). These are available in a free

Table 1.2: Distribution of values, lower reference limits, and their 95% CI for semen parameters from fertile men those partners had a time-to-time pregnancy of 12 months or less.

Seminal parameter	95% CI
• Volume	1.5 milliliters
• pH	7.2
• Concentration	15 million spermatozoa per milliliter
• Total number of spermatozoa	39 million spermatozoa per ejaculation
• Motility	40% total motility (progressive + nonprogressive) 32% progressive motility
• Vitality	58% spermatozoa alive per ejaculation
• Morphology	4% normal shape

access article published in May 2010 in *Human Reproduction Update,*[12] offering, with more clarity, lower reference limits of the fifth percentile of the values for a fertile male reference population.

This is accompanied by some changes in the samples diagnosis. Therefore, despite maintaining the nomenclature, there are some changes:

- *Teratozoospermia*: Normal shape by strict criteria (Tygerberg) <4%
- *Asthenozoospermia*: PM <32% does not take into account total motility (% PR + NP) even if under the reference value.
- *Oligozoospermia*: Total number of spermatozoa <39 million. The WHO prefers this parameter to sample concentration, which was the selectable parameter in the Manual of 1999.
- *Necrozoospermia*: Vitality <58% and very high IM percentage. The second criterion is arbitrary since the WHO does not specify a number, but it does talk about much IM. This way, fake necrozoospermia, which can alarm unjustifiably, is avoided.
- *Cryptozoospermia/azoospermia*: There are no changes from 1999.

PROBLEMS AND IMPROVEMENTS OF THE NEW WHO CLASSIFICATION

As it occurs in every change or review, we have found not only significant improvements but also some issues that we will need to solve as we get familiarized with the modifications. Some of these issues were as follows:

- New concept of oligozoospermia. In 1999, the WHO assigned this diagnosis to those samples with concentration under the reference value of this parameter (20 million/mL). However, it has become clear that this concentration depends on the final volume of the sample. That is the reason why the manual of 2010 links preferably the oligozoospermia diagnosis to the total number of spermatozoa, provided that it is under 39 million. This is an improvement in the assessment of this parameter.

- New categories of sperm motility. The old category "a" from the manual of 1999 was difficult to justify without a computerized system to count motility in the sample. It was actually observed that the relevant information from this parameter was in the total number of PM (a + b). For these two reasons, sperm motility categories were modified. Now, it is recommended to differentiate spermatozoa in three categories or types: PM, NP, and IM. Some centers consider the new classification as an advantage.

- Decrease of the percentage of normal shapes in morphology analysis. It is well known that this is not only the most subjective parameter of the semen analysis but also the one which creates the most controversy when choosing one treatment type or another in assisted reproduction clinics. Numerous articles have been published for and against the importance of morphology in many key aspects of these treatments: pregnancy rate, implantation rate, fertilization success, etc.[13-17] Anyway, it has always been debated not only in andrology and IVF laboratories but also between these departments and the clinical departments. This is due to the fact that, apart from extreme morphology cases with many anomalies, it is difficult to unify morphological assessment criteria to evaluate the samples, even when performing the appropriate internal and external quality assurances.

- Sperm vitality and necrozoospermia. It looks like this parameter, not included in the WHO as a "compulsory study" in the seminogram but as something very advisable, is gaining importance in this new edition. Because this parameter is linked to the percentage of sperm IM but there is not an exact fixed value from which necrozoospermia can be diagnosed, each group can decide that value individually depending on the methodology employed in their center and the information expected from the diagnosis. It is well known that the vitality study is essential in those cases with a percentage of sperm IM over 50%. It is not the same to have a high percentage of immotile spermatozoa that are alive after the stain test, which would guide toward possible structural flaws in the tail,[18] than a high percentage of immotile spermatozoa which are also dead, more related to an epididymis pathology.[19,20]

- The disappearance of the "adjectives" mild, moderate, and severe results in diagnosis of the samples being incomplete and obliges to take into account numerical values of volume, concentration, motility, and morphology to get a real idea of the state of the sample. Depending on the number of millions of progressive motile spermatozoa, each center or laboratory, can decide the type of treatment for a couple.

Table 1.3: Different male seminogram reference values and parameters in 1999 and 2010.

Seminal parameter	Semen 1999	Semen 2010
• Volume	2.0 milliliters	1.5 milliliters
• Concentration	20×10^6 spermatozoa per milliliter	15×10^6 spermatozoa per milliliter 39×10^6 total spermatozoa
• Progressive motility	50%	32%
• Morphology	15% normal shape	4% normal shape
• Millions of progressive motile	20	7.2 12

- Finally, the most remarkable aspect is probably the different male semi-nogram reference values and parameters in 1999 and 2010. In Table 1.3, a comparison of the two possible situations is described.

As it can be observed, the number of millions of progressive motile spermatozoa is reduced by 64%—or 40% if we use the total spermatozoa criterion that is now advised—to the number obtained for a semen sample of a male according to the reference values of 1999. The change of this aspect could cause more problems at clinical consultation level, since males now diagnosed as normal may still receive the recommendation to be submitted to an intrauterine insemination (IUI) or even an IVF cycle. Obviously, each center should decide whether they change their criteria or they explain to every patient that with the current reference values there is the possibility that, even being "normal", they could have subfertility that would need a specific-assisted reproduction treatment.

DEBATE

First of all, it is important to remember that the seminogram does not have diagnosis capacity per se—sensitivity and specificity—to indicate male infertility. Seminogram diagnosis are better understood merely as a sample description to check that they "are similar" to the values of a fertile popula-tion. Nonetheless, they could be useful in the clinical diagnosis to detect cryptozoospermia or azoospermia.

On the other hand, for people who work in assisted reproduction it is important to differentiate between the male seminal diagnosis and the "real" use of the sample in an infertility treatment. We know that WHO establishes clearly that being under the reference values or having a sample not "normozoospermic" does not necessarily mean male infertility but it shows that seminal parameter is under the fifth percentile in a reference population of fertile males, i.e. it means that this value is under 95% of the values presented by these fertile males. Theoretically, it is likely that the reference values keep on updating as population studies get widened, especially due to the way those values were obtained—statistics of parameters in 2,000 fertile male. Apart from its utility for the diagnosis of an infertile couple, the seminogram is, together with the other tests and examinations, a useful tool to make therapeutic decisions. Its main goal is to evaluate if the sample, once prepared, allows obtaining the minimum number of millions of progressive motile spermatozoa to follow one reproduction treatment or another: artificial insemination or IUI, in vitro fertilization or IVF, or intracytoplasmic sperm injection (ICSI). We could think that for standard IVF the new reference values should not modify the internal values established by every laboratory according to their insemination protocols. However, we should be careful with normozoospermic samples containing values under the lower limits of the different parameters, as aforementioned. Finally, morphology determination is still a parameter with doubtful clinical utility to recommend a patient directly to IVF or ICSI treatment, and therefore should be considered with caution.

REFERENCES

1. World Health Organization. WHO Laboratory Manual for the Examination of Human Semen and Sperm-Cervical Mucus Interaction, 4th edition. Cambridge: Cambridge University Press; 1999. 128pp.
2. World Health Organization. Sperm Collection and Processing Methods. Cambridge: Cambridge University Press; 1999.
3. World Health Organization. WHO Manual for the Standardized Investigation and Diagnosis of the Infertile Male. Cambridge: Cambridge University Press; 1999.
4. Cooper TG, Neuwinger J, Bahrs S, et al. Internal quality control of semen analysis. Fertil Steril. 1992;58:172-8.
5. Dunphy BC, Kay R, Barratt CL, et al. Quality control during the conventional analysis of semen, an essential exercise. J Androl. 1989;10:378-85.
6. Neuwinger J, Behre HM, Nieschlag E. External quality control in the andrology laboratory: an experimental multicenter trial. Fertil Steril. 1990;54:308-14.
7. Comhaire FH, Vermeulen L, Schoonjans F. Reassessment of the accuracy of traditional sperm characteristics and adenosine triphosphate (ATP) in estimating the fertilizing potential of human semen in vivo. Int J Androl. 1987;10:653-62.
8. Ombelet W, Bosmans E, Janssen M, et al. Semen parameters in a fertile versus subfertile population: a need for change in the interpretation of semen testing. Hum Reprod. 1997;12:987-93.
9. Ombelet W, Wouters E, Bolees L, et al. Sperm morphology assessment: diagnostic potential and comparative analysis of strict or WHO criteria in a fertile and subfertile population. Int J Androl. 1997;20:367-72.
10. Castilla JA, Alvarez C, Aguilar J, et al. Influence of analytical and biological variation on the clinical interpretation of seminal parameters. Hum Reprod. 2006;21:847-51.

11. Cooper TG, Yeung CH. Computer-aided evaluation of assessment of "grade a" spermatozoa by experienced technicians. Fertil Steril. 2006;85:220-24.
12. Cooper TG, Noonan E, von Eckardstein S, et al. World Health Organization reference values for human semen characteristics. Hum Reprod Update. 2010; 16(3):231-45.
13. Kruger TF, Menkveld R, Stander FS, et al. Sperm morphologic features as a prognostic factor in vitro fertilization. Fertil Steril. 1986;46:1118-23.
14. Kruger TF, Acosta AA, Simmons KF, et al. Predictive value of abnormal sperm morphology in vitro fertilization. Fertil Steril. 1988;49:112-17.
15. Menkveld R, Stander FSH, Kotze TJ, et al. The evaluation of morphological characteristics of human spermatozoa according to stricter criteria. Hum Reprod. 1990;5(5):586-92.
16. Mortimer D, Menkveld R. Sperm morphology assessment. Historical perspectives and current opinions. J Androl. 2001;22:192-205.
17. Garrido N, Meseguer M, Martínez-Conejero JA, et al. Impacto de los criterios estrictos de morfología espermática en reproducción Asistida. Cuadernos de Medicina Reproductiva, Vol. 11, No. 1. Año 2005.
18. Chemes HE, Rawe VY. Sperm pathology: a step beyond descriptive morphology. Origin, characterization and fertility potential of abnormal sperm phenotypes in infertile men. Hum Reprod Update. 2003;9:405-28.
19. Wilton LJ, Temple-Smith PD, Baker HWG, et al. Human male infertility caused by degeneration and death of sperm in the epididymis. Fertil Steril. 1988;49: 1052-58.
20. Correa-Pérez JR, Fernández-Pelegrina R, Aslanis P, et al. Clinical management of men producing ejaculates characterized by high levels of dead sperm and altered seminal plasma factors consistent with epididymal necrospermia. Fert Steril. 2004;81(4):1148-50.

CHAPTER 2

Investigating the Subfertile Male: Which Tests are Practically Relevant?

Alberto Pacheco Castro, Cristina González Ravina

INTRODUCTION

Male infertility is directly or indirectly responsible for 50% of the cases involving fertility-related failures in reproductive couples. Since intracytoplasmic sperm injection (ICSI) into oocytes was described, most of these cases have been treated with this procedure, especially when that failure is due to severe male factor infertility.[1,2] However, current success rates of this procedure remain suboptimal. The reason for this is that current diagnoses of male factor infertility are mainly based on sperm parameters of concentration, motility, viability, and morphology. Also, nowadays, selection of sperm during ICSI is mainly based on motility and morphology.[3] These criteria are clearly inadequate to detect abnormalities at a molecular level, which may have a negative impact on pregnancy rate. Invisible anomalies such as intracellular oxidative stress, externalization of plasma membrane phosphatidylserine, disruption of mitochondrial membrane potential and, more importantly, damaged chromatin are barely taken into account.[4]

In a large number of reproductive centers, male factor is only determined by an anamnesis and a semen profile. Indeed, male factor infertility is usually defined in terms of conventional semen analysis, where descriptive information is only given concerning the number of spermatozoa present in the ejaculate sample and the proportion of them which are motile or morphologically normal and related to "normal" threshold values established by World Health Organization.[5]

Thus, when conventional seminal study confirms a serious defect, especially at the level of sperm concentration (<5 million/mL), supplementary studies are required to improve the diagnosis, especially in order to determine genetic or chromosomal abnormalities. Among them, the most desirable (apart from karyotype analysis) are (a) study of chromosomal alterations by fluorescence in situ hybridization assay, (b) study of prevalent genetic mutations, e.g. cystic fibrosis, and (c) analysis of Y-chromosome microdeletions. Depending on the results, the clinician can evaluate the possibility of carrying out an assisted reproduction technique (ART) or performing a complementary technique (preimplantation genetic diagnosis). However, if the risk of transmitting genetic disorders to the offspring is high, or if the probabilities of a successful treatment are very low, the clinician should consider the suitability of a change of male gamete for the ART.

However, a high proportion of patients attending clinics present normal values or only moderate defects in sperm analysis. In most cases, no additional tests are performed in these subfertile or "normal" individuals. It is important to mention that normal reference values for semen parameters do not equate with the minimum values required for pregnancy. *Patients with semen variables outside the reference ranges may be fertile and, conversely, men with values within the reference range may still be infertile.* Clearly, in such cases, conventional semen analysis has been unable to identify the functional defects responsible for infertility,[6] indicating that if the only evaluation made on the patient is a semen analysis, then an underlying pathology can be missed.

In the past decade, several methods have been developed to improve diagnosis of male subfertility. Many of them have been shown to exhibit prognostic utility that eluded the conventional semen analysis. As a consequence, nowadays, we have new tools to investigate the functional capacity of sperm and, if necessary, to separate spermatozoa through other parameters different from the motility as used in conventional separation methods. In this chapter, several of them will be discussed, highlighting the laboratory methods available to assess these aspects of sperm structure and function and focusing on their clinical application.

SPERM DNA FRAGMENTATION

DNA integrity is one of the most important elements of sperm quality and it correlates not only with impaired pregnancy rates in vivo and in vitro but also with the health and well-being of the offspring.[7]

DNA damage can be a consequence of many different factors: drugs, pollution, alcohol, smoking, increased testicular temperature, infections, varicocele, male age, or genetic lesions.

Although the main role of sperm DNA integrity is well known[8] and it is also established that abnormal DNA damage is more frequent in infertile patients,[9] there is considerable controversy about the possible diagnostic and/or prognostic value of the tests currently used to study sperm DNA fragmentation. This can be due to several factors:
- *Origin of DNA damage:* There are different mechanisms by which DNA can be damaged: defective sperm chromatin condensation during

maturation, apoptosis,[10] oxidative stress[11] and genetic lesions.[12] This damage may originate from intrinsic (changes in spermatogenesis, genetic causes) or extrinsic (genital infections) factors, and maybe interdependent between them.

- *Types of sperm DNA damage:* There are two types of DNA strand breaks: single- and double-stranded breaks. These breaks could develop from different clinical causes. Double-stranded breaks are less capable of being repaired by the oocyte than single-stranded breaks. They indicate more profound defects and clinical implications.
- *Sperm DNA fragmentation tests:* There are many different clinical tests (Table 2.1) used to analyze sperm DNA fragmentation, among which: (a) single-cell gel electrophoresis assay (COMET),[9] (b) sperm chromatin structure assay (SCSA),[13] (c) terminal deoxynucleotidyl transferase-mediated dUTP Nick End Labeling (TUNEL),[14] and (d) alkaline gel electrophoresis,[15] or sperm chromatin decondensation (SCD) test. These tests have different cutoff values (20% for TUNEL assay, 30% for SCSA) and the results obtained from them do not exactly correlate in some cases, suggesting that all tests do not analyze the same level of DNA damage.

Clinical Applications of Sperm DNA Fragmentation

The study of sperm DNA fragmentation would be especially useful in (a) older patients (> 45 years old), (b) patients with "normal" seminal parameters

Table 2.1: Main sperm DNA fragmentation tests.

Test	Author/year	Mechanism analyzed	Pretreatment	Technique of analysis
TUNEL	Gorczyca et al.[16] (1993)	Incorporation of fluorescent labeled dUTP by tdt enzyme	No	Fluorescence microscopy or cytometry
SCSA	Evenson et al.[17] (1995)	Metachromatic properties of acridine orange with single- and double-stranded DNA	Yes (acid)	Cytometry
COMET	Aitken et al.[18] (1998)	Differences of single- and double-stranded DNA migration in an electric field	No	Electrophoresis
SCD	Fernandez et al.[19] (2002)	Differences on release of DNA loops	Yes (acid)	Microscopy

(TUNEL: Deoxynucleotidyl transferase-mediated dUTP nick end labeling assay; SCSA: Sperm Chromatin stability assay; COMET: Single-cell electrophoresis assay; SCD: Sperm chromatin decondensation assay).

or slight alterations but long duration infertility (>3 years), and (c) patients with severe seminal alterations but no genetic anomalies.

Since there is a strong correlation between sperm DNA fragmentation and miscarriage,[20] other relevant candidates for this study are couples with previous failures using ART without known female factor and cases of recurrent miscarriages.

More importantly, this analysis of sperm DNA damage will enable us to obtain significant functional sperm quality data. However, it does not explain the origin of functional alteration. Thus, the best approach would be performing the DNA fragmentation test and other functional tests (such as H3 oxidative stress and H4 apoptosis) to help us determine the source of the damage and/or take a different clinical approach (reduction of sexual abstinence, antioxidant therapy, selection of nonapoptotic spermatozoa).

OXIDATIVE STRESS

Sperm oxidative status is crucial to spermatozoa functionality.[21] Human spermatozoa are particularly sensitive to oxidative stress due to their high cellular content of polyunsaturated fatty acids, together with a defective natural antioxidant defense capacity.[22] Indeed, oxidative stress created by excessive generation of reactive oxygen species (ROS) and/or impairment of antioxidant protection within the male reproductive tract[7] can cause damage in the plasma membrane (lipid peroxidation) and in the mitochondrial function as well as a disruption of cell functionality. Finally, this triggers alterations in sperm DNA integrity and results in cell death by apoptotic processes. Under physiological conditions, these spermatozoa are retained in the female reproductive tract and never reach the oocyte. But when experts are working with the sample in the laboratory, this selection process does not occur correctly and, as a result, the spermatozoa with less functionality can be used for ART.

At present, there are several methods to analyze sperm oxidative stress, which have advantages and disadvantages. Historically, the most commonly used method has been the chemiluminescence analysis. But the main problem with this technique is that the measurement obtained may be contaminated by oxidative stress produced by leukocytes, cells with much greater power for ROS generation. Therefore, it is essential to eliminate the cells which may contain some magnetic particles having anti-CD45 (leukocyte cell-specific) antibodies. An alternative technique uses certain lipophilic fluorescent compounds that give us a direct measure of cellular oxidative status. Among them, the most used are DHE, DCFH, and 8-hydroxy guanosine. Nonetheless, in order to accomplish these steps, a flow cytometer is needed so that the results obtained are representative and consistent.

Oxidative stress can also be analyzed by determining the cellular lipid peroxidation.[23] In these cases, the most common tests are the ones that determine malonaldehyde by ELISA and the analysis of lipid peroxidation by flow cytometry using BODIPY compound.[24] Finally, another commonly used analysis focuses on determining sperm DNA fragmentation through different techniques. This analysis is also a good procedure, somehow related indirectly to the oxidative status, therefore correlating oxidative status and sperm functional capacity.[8]

Clinical Application of Oxidative Stress Analysis: Antioxidant Therapy

Today, there are several products in the market with antioxidant properties to improve sperm oxidative status and, as a result, to improve the semen quality (increasing its concentration and improving sperm motility). Among them, the most commonly used are Selenium, Vitamin C, Vitamin E, and zinc.[25] Not only do they improve semen parameters but also these compounds can help improve other functional characteristics (Table 2.2) of sperm and, thus, they help to increase pregnancy rates in infertile couples. Indeed, a recent Cochrane meta-analysis about the use of oral antioxidant in cases of male infertility found that these agents significantly improve pregnancy rates and live birth rates.[26] Interestingly, in this analysis, a significant decrease of sperm DNA damage was also found after 2–3 months of antioxidant therapy, but improvements in semen parameters were not evident, suggesting that these treatments improve functional capability of spermatozoa rather than testicular function. However, more studies are needed to confirm these promising results.

SPERM APOPTOSIS

It is well known that apoptosis plays an important role in the regulation of spermatogenesis. It implies the induction of a series of cellular and

Table 2.2: Compounds commonly used as antioxidant properties in oral antioxidant therapy.

Compound	Sperm functional properties
• Selenium	• Reduces lipid peroxidation
• Vitamin E	• Improves cell and mitochondrial membrane integrity
• Vitamin C	• Scavenger of oxidative species molecules, reduces DNA fragmentation
• Q10 coenzyme	• Improves of cell membrane integrity, reduces DNA fragmentation
• Zinc	• Reduces sperm oxidative stress and sperm DNA fragmentation
• Lycopene	• Reduces sperm DNA fragmentation

biochemical changes that lead the cell to commit suicide without eliciting an inflammatory response.[27] Apoptosis is based on a genetic mechanism, whose main objective is to control the overproduction of spermatozoa, restricting it to normal levels of proliferation. Tests show that germ cell apoptosis occurs during spermatogenesis, mainly in spermatogonia and the meiotic cell division. This generates excessive breakage of chromatin and increased DNA fragmentation. Indeed, multiple studies have established that in patients diagnosed with male infertility, the proportion of apoptotic sperm in ejaculated semen samples is higher.[28,29] Several studies have studied the relationship between seminal parameters and apoptosis in ejaculated semen. A significant negative correlation between the proportion of apoptotic cells and sperm viability and motility in ejaculated semen has been reported.[29-31]

Mature sperm cells have been reported to express distinct markers of apoptosis-related cell damage.[27,32,33] One of the earlier markers is the externalization of phosphatidylserine (EPS) residues to the sperm outer membrane leaflet. Nevertheless, it is not clear whether the apoptotic markers detected in spermatozoa are residues of an abortive apoptotic process started before ejaculation or whether they result from apoptosis initiated in the postejaculation period.[27,34,35]

In order to select nonapoptotic spermatozoa fraction and improve sperm preparation protocols for ICSI, a new sperm selection technique called MACS has been described (magnetic-activated cell sorting). This technique is based on the EPS to the outer surface of the sperm membrane in apoptotic sperm. This allows its binding with annexin-V-conjugated paramagnetic microbeads, which could be used to label and separate apoptotic spermatozoa using a magnetic-activated cell sorting system.[36] A heterogeneous sperm cell suspension is incubated with annexin-V-conjugated microbeads, which bind to only apoptotic sperm with EPS. Then, the bead/sperm mixture is allowed to run through the MACS column, which is placed inside a magnet. The magnetic force will cause the retention of the cells labeled with microbeads inside the column, while the nonlabeled cells will flow freely.

OTHER FUNCTIONAL TESTS

There are a series of functional tests that have been employed mainly in research studies, although some of them may be used for the diagnosis of male infertility in the near future. One of the more promising tests is the analysis of acrosome reaction of human sperm induced by different agents (calcium ionophore or progesterone). Also, the measurement of different biochemical markers such as sperm creatine kinase or Catsperm function may be of interest in the improvement of male diagnosis. But currently these tests have a limited role, because they have little proven clinical utility.

CONCLUSION

Determination of reliable and accurate methods to study the fertilizing potential of sperm is of vital importance to provide a definitive diagnosis of the underlying causes of idiopathic male fertility. Identifying the exact nature of the defect will help select the appropriate procedures, which in turn will improve natural and assisted reproduction success rates and help ensure healthy offspring. This may also help identify the group of men and their offspring that, through techniques such as ICSI, may propagate their genetic complement linked to male infertility.

REFERENCES

1. Sherins RJ, Thorsell LP, Dorfmann A, et al. Intracytoplasmic sperm injection facilitates fertilization even in the most severe forms of male infertility: pregnancy outcome correlates with maternal age and number of eggs available. Fert Ster. 1995; 64:369-75.
2. Jain T, Gupta RS. Trends in the use of intracytoplasmic sperm injection in the United States. N Engl J Med. 2007;357:251-7.
3. Henkel RR, Schill WB. Sperm preparation for ART. Reprod Biol Endocrinol. 2003;1:108.
4. Zhang HB, Lu SM, Ma CY, et al. Early apoptotic changes in human spermatozoa and their relationships with conventional semen parameters and sperm DNA fragmentation. Asian J Androl. 2008;10:227-35.
5. World Health Organization. WHO Laboratory Manual for the Examination of Human Semen and Sperm-Cervical Mucus Interaction, 5th edition. Cambridge: Cambridge University Press;2010.
6. Nallela KP, Sharma RK, Aziz N, et al. Significance of sperm characteristics in the evaluation of male infertility. Fert Ster. 2006;85(3):629-34.
7. Aitken RJ, Bennetts LE, Sawyer D, et al. Impact of radio frequency electromagnetic radiation on DNA integrity in the male germline. Int J Androl. 2005;28(3):171-9.
8. Lewis S, Aitken RJ. DNA damage to spermatozoa has impacts on fertilization and pregnancy. Cell Tissue Res. 2005;322:33-41.
9. Irvine DS, Twigg JP, Gordon EL, et al. DNA integrity in human spermatozoa: relationships with semen quality. J Androl. 2000;21:33-44.
10. Shen H, Ong C. Detection of oxidative DNA damage in human sperm and its association with sperm function and male infertility. Free Radic Biol Med. 2000;28:529-36.
11. Said TM, Aziz N, Sharma RK, et al. Novel association between sperm deformity index and oxidative stress-induced DNA damage in infertile male patients. Asian J Androl. 2005;7:121-6.
12. Sharma RK, Said T, Agarwal A. Sperm DNA damage and its clinical relevance in assessing reproductive outcome. Asian J Androl. 2004;6:139-48.
13. Evenson DP, Jost LK, Marshall D, et al. Utility of the sperm chromatin structure assay as a diagnostic and prognostic tool in the human fertility clinic. Hum Reprod. 1999;14(4):1039-49.
14. Sun JG, Jurisicova A, Casper RF. Detection of deoxyribonucleic acid fragmentation in human sperm: correlation with fertilization in vitro. Biol Reprod. 1997;56:602-7.

15. Sawyer DE, Mercer BG, Wiklendt AM, et al. Quantitative analysis of gene-specific DNA damage in human spermatozoa. Mutat Res. 2003;529(1):21-34.

16. Gorczyca W, Traganos F, Jesionowska H, et al. Presence of DNA strand breaks and increased sensitivity of DNA in situ to denaturation in abnormal human sperm cells: analogy to apoptosis of somatic cells. Exp Cell Res 1993;207:202-5.

17. Evenson D, Jost L, Gandour D, et al. Comparative sperm chromatin structure assay measurements on epiillumination and orthogonal axes flow cytometers. Cytometry 1995;19:295-303.

18. Aitken RJ, Gordon E, Harkiss D. et al. Relative Impact of Oxidative Stress on the Functional Competence and Genomic Integrity of Human Spermatozoa. Biol Reprod 1998;59:1037-46.

19. Fernández JL, Muriel L, Rivero MT. et al. The sperm chromatin dispersion test: a simple method for the determination of sperm DNA fragmentation. J Androl. 2003;24:59-66.

20. Robinson L, Gallos ID, Conner SJ, et al. The effect of sperm DNA fragmentation on miscarriage rates: a systematic review and meta-analysis. Hum Reprod. 2012;27(10):2908-17.

21. Henkel RR. Leukocytes and oxidative stress: dilemma for sperm function and male fertility. Asian J Androl. 2011;13(1):43-52.

22. Aitken RJ, Baker MA. Oxidative stress, sperm survival and fertility control. Mol Cell Endocrin. 2006;250(1):66-9.

23. Gomez E, Irvine DS, Aitken RJ. Evaluation of a spectrophotometric assay for the measurement of malondialdehyde and 4-hydroxyalkenals in human spermatozoa: relationships with semen quality and sperm function. Int J Androl. 1998;21:81-94.

24. Aitken RJ, Wingate J, de Iuliis GN, et al. Analysis of lipid peroxidation in human spermatozoa using BODIPY C11. Mol Hum Reprod. 2007;13:203-11.

25. Ross C, Morriss A, Khairy M, et al. A systematic review of the effect of oral antioxidants on male infertility. RBM Online. 2010;20(6):711-23.

26. Showell MG, Brown J, Yazdani A, et al. Antioxidants for male subfertility. Cochrane Database Syst Rev. 2011;(1):CD007411.

27. Grunewald S, Paasch U, Wuendrich K, et al. Sperm caspases become more activated in infertility patients than in healthy donors during cryopreservation. Syst Biol Reprod Med. 2005;51(6):449-60.

28. Sakkas D, Seli E, Bizzaro D, et al. Abnormal spermatozoa in the ejaculate: abortive apoptosis and faulty nuclear remodelling during spermatogenesis. RBM Online. 2003;7:428-32.

29. Taylor SL, Weng SL, Fox P, et al. Somatic cell apoptosis markers and pathways in human ejaculated sperm: potential utility as indicators of sperm quality. Mol Hum Reprod. 2004;10(11):825-34.

30. Marchetti C, Obert G, Deffosez A, et al. Study of mitochondrial membrane potential, reactive oxygen species, DNA fragmentation and cell viability by flow cytometry in human sperm. Hum Reprod. 2002;17:1257-65.

31. Said TM, Grunewald S, Paasch U, et al. Effects of magnetic-activated cell sorting on sperm motility and cryosurvival rates. Fert Ster. 2005;83:1442-6.

32. Muratori M, Piomboni P, Baldi E, et al. Functional and ultrastructural features of DNA-fragmented human sperm. J Androl. 2000;21(6):903-12.

33. Shen HM, Dai J, Chia SE, et al. Detection of apoptotic alterations in sperm in subfertile patients and their correlations with sperm quality. Hum Reprod. 2002;17(5):1266-73.

34. Tesarik J. Paternal effects on cell division in the preimplantation embryo. RBM Online. 2005;10(3):370-75.
35. Lachaud C, Tesarik J, Cañadas ML, et al. Apoptosis and necrosis in human ejaculated spermatozoa. Hum Reprod. 2004;19(3):607-10.
36. Lee TH, Liu CH, Shih YT, et al. Magnetic-activated cell sorting for sperm preparation reduces spermatozoa with apoptotic markers and improves the acrosome reaction in couples with unexplained infertility. Hum Reprod. 2010;25:839-46.

CHAPTER
3

Managing Ejaculation Failure

Rupin Shah

INTRODUCTION

Failure to ejaculate is a relatively uncommon, and therefore poorly understood, cause of infertility, and can prove be a major stumbling block during infertility treatment. In this chapter, we outline a practical approach to the diagnosis and management of this problem.

Failure to ejaculate may be situational or total. In *situational anejaculation*, the man is able to ejaculate under some circumstances but not in others. In *total anejaculation*, the man never ejaculates during intercourse or masturbation.

Situational anejaculation occurs due to psychological reasons. No investigations are needed. Therapy is focused on strategies to anticipate and prevent the problem, and to obtain a semen sample if the problem does occur.

Total anejaculation may occur because a man never reaches conscious orgasm and therefore does not ejaculate—*anorgasmic anejaculation*, or may occur despite a man reaching an orgasm—*orgasmic anejaculation*. Anorgasmic anejaculation occurs due to psychological or physiological reasons, while orgasmic anejaculation is always due to a physical defect—usually anatomical or neurological.[1]

SITUATIONAL ANEJACULATION

There are various types of situational anejaculation. The diagnosis is obvious from history and no investigations are needed. The various types of situational anejaculation, and strategies for their prevention and management, are discussed below:

- *Unexpected failure of ejaculation*: This happens to a man who has had no problem giving a semen sample in the past but suddenly, unexpectedly, fails to give a sample on the day of IUI or OPU during an IVF cycle. This happens due to the stress of the infertility treatment and the pressure of having to give a sample under such conditions. This can happen to anyone and so the best preventive measure is to cryopreserve a sample in advance for all IVF couples. If that has not been done, a semen sample may be obtained by the use of a vibrator or electroejaculation, or sperm can be aspirated from the testis and used for ICSI.

- *Periovulatory anejaculation/on-demand anejaculation*: In this situation, the man has difficulty in collecting a semen sample at the time of ovulation, when he is under pressure to perform, though he is able to ejaculate easily at other times. Sometimes, the infertility specialist contributes to the problem by giving a specific time of ovulation so that the wife wakes up the husband at 4 AM to have sex at the right time!! This treatment-induced sexual dysfunction can be minimized by giving the couple a fertile period and emphasizing that they can have sex during this period as per their inclination and pleasure. Some men will benefit from the use of an erectogenic drug like sildenafil that can be given in a dose of 50 mg, one hour before intercourse, and is safe for conception. In refractory cases, a vibrator may be used to get a semen sample that can be used for IUI.

- *Clinic anejaculation*: A fair number of men, who can ejaculate easily at home, find it difficult to ejaculate in the clinic because they become self-conscious and feel under pressure. This problem can be avoided by ensuring that the semen collection room is discretely placed, is clean, and has a bed so that the couple can be together, if required. Sometimes providing erotic material will help. If the problem has been identified during the sexual history at the initial interview (these questions should be part of standard fertility history) then the man can be allowed to bring the sample from home. Otherwise, most men with this problem can ejaculate in the clinic with the help of a vibrator.

- *Masturbation anejaculation*: Some men are unaccustomed to masturbation and are unable to give a sample by manipulation even though they ejaculate during intercourse. Therefore, when asking a man to produce a semen sample it is always important to check whether he will be able to produce a sample by masturbation in the clinic. If he expresses his inability to do so he can be asked to collect a sample at home by coitus interruptus.

- *Intercourse anejaculation*: In this condition, a man can ejaculate during masturbation but not by intercourse. The cause is usually psychogenic or technical (lack of adequate stimulation). Treatment is through sex therapy and counseling but is often difficult. Fertility can be easily achieved by IUI used the masturbatory sample.

ANORGASMIC ANEJACULATION

In this condition, the man does not ejaculate because he never reaches an orgasm, either during intercourse or during masturbation.

The etiology may be:
- *Psychological*: Due to early negative sexual experiences or strict, inhibitory religious upbringing
- *Technical*: Due to inadequate stimulation during intercourse due to poor erections or improper intercourse
- *Physiological*: Due to a high ejaculatory threshold (the opposite of premature ejaculation). This seems to be the commonest cause in our patients
- *Pharmacological*: Due to antipsychotics that can cause marked inhibition and delay of orgasm.
- *Neurological*: Due to reduced glans sensation or dorsal nerve neuropathy.

Diagnosis is based on the history alone and usually does not need investigations. Classically, the man gives a history of prolonged intercourse without reaching an orgasm, and finally stopping because he is tired. However, a man who has never experienced orgasm is often unclear about whether he has reached an orgasm or not, and hence the history may be unclear. Many of these men will, however, state that they though do not ejaculate during intercourse they have spontaneous ejaculations at night. *A history of nocturnal emissions is very important because it rules out an organic cause of anejaculation.*

Treatment through psychosexual therapy may help in some cases but is time-consuming and frequently unfruitful. When the primary concern is fertility (rather than orgasm and sexual pleasure) then more active measures to obtain sperm by vibrator stimulation[2] or electroejaculation[3,4] should be tried right away.

ORGASMIC ANEJACULATION

These men reach an orgasm but do not ejaculate. The cause is always organic.

When a man reaches a climax the orgasm is usually accompanied by ejaculation that occurs in three phases:
- *Phase 1 (emission)*: Stimulation of the sympathetic fibers causes the seminal vesicles, prostate, vasa, and tails of the epididymides to contract and deposit seminal fluid into the posterior urethra.
- *Phase 2 (bladder neck closure)*: Simultaneously, again under sympathetic control, the bladder neck closes to prevent retrograde ejaculation.
- *Phase 3 (antegrade propulsion)*: Seminal fluid flows from the posterior into the bulbar urethra. Rhythmic contractions of the bulbocavernosus muscle propel the fluid out of the urethra with forceful squirts.

Any of these three phases can be affected by anatomical, neurogenic, or pharmacological factors resulting in orgasmic anejaculation. Some of the common causes are listed below:

- *Phase 1 disorder (anatomical)*: Ductal obstruction due to genitourinary Kocks
- *Phase 1 disorder (neurogenic)*: Spinal cord injury; lumbar sympathectomy; pelvic surgery; RPLND; diabetic neuropathy; α-adrenergic blockers
- *Phase 1 disorder (endocrine)*: Severe hypogonadism (very low testosterone) due to primary or secondary testicular failure
- *Phase 2 disorder (anatomical)*: Bladder neck disruption due to bladder neck trauma (fracture pelvis), bladder neck incision (iatrogenic), or congenitally wide bladder neck
- *Phase 2 disorder (neurogenic)*: Diabetic neuropathy; α-adrenergic blockers
- *Phase 3 disorder (anatomical)*: Outflow obstruction due to stricture, diverticulum or urethral pouch; damage to the bulbocavernosus muscle during urethral reconstruction
- *Phase 3 disorder (neurogenic)*: Paralysis of the bulbocavernosus muscle.

Diagnosis is frequently possible from history alone. Retrograde ejaculation is diagnosed by examination of the postorgasm urine for sperm.

Treatment depends on etiology. Neurogenic failure of emission or retrograde ejaculation due to neuropathy may respond to a 10-day course of a combination of a sympathomimetic (ephedrine 30 mg TDS; pseudoephedrine 60 mg TDS) and an anticholinergic (imipramine 25 mg 2HS).[5] Other cases of neurogenic failure can be treated with vibrator stimulation or electroejaculation.[6] In men with spinal cord injury success will depend on the spinal level of the lesion.[7] RPLND usually results in failure of ejaculation rather than retrograde ejaculation; semen can be obtained by electroejaculation.[8]

Anatomical obstruction causing failure of emission is usually too extensive to be corrected by endoscopic surgery and the only option is epididymal or testicular sperm aspiration and ICSI.

Retrograde ejaculation due to diabetic neuropathy may respond to medical therapy as above. Otherwise sperm can be retrieved from the bladder and used for IUI or ICSI depending on the quality. When sperm is being retrieved from the bladder the urine must be made alkaline and dilute to improve sperm survival. Accordingly the patient is given a urinary alkalizer (soda bicarb or potassium citrate thrice a day) for 3 days. On the day of retrieval, he consumes three glasses of water with the alkalizer and then passes urine every 30 minutes. The urine pH is checked each time and when it is above 7.5 the man masturbates and then immediately voids urine. This is quickly centrifuged to separate the sperm; the sperm pellet is then rewashed with medium and used for IUI. If the motility of the recovered sperm is poor then an alternative method is to instill 30 mL of sperm-washing medium in the bladder and then ask the man to masturbate.

When there is failure of antegrade propulsion the semen will dribble out later. This can be collected and used for IUI or IVF. In all cases of orgasmic anejaculation, if other measures fail, sperm retrieval from the testes and ICSI is the final solution.

VIBRATOR THERAPY

This is extremely useful in treating situational anejaculation, anorgasmic anejaculation, and some cases of neurogenic orgasmic anejaculation.

The vibrator works by strongly stimulating the afferent pathways of the ejaculatory reflex. This overcomes inhibition due to situational, psychological, or neurogenic factors, thus resulting in orgasm and ejaculation.

The patient is prepared for the vibrator by counseling him that the ejaculation will happen automatically and that he should *not try* to ejaculate. This will allow him to be relaxed and will reduce cortical inhibition of ejaculation due to anxiety. It also helps avoid pseudoejaculation of urine that happens when a nonorgasmic man strains to ejaculate.

He then sits on a bed in a quiet room and self-stimulates and fantasizes to achieve some tumescence. A full erection is not mandatory and the patient is reassured that he would be able to ejaculate even if he does not have an erection. If the man is very anxious then an anxiolytic and PDE5 inhibitor may be given. The vibrator is then positioned so that the undersurface of the glans penis rests upon the vibrating head. Gentle pressure is applied to the penis so that maximum vibration is felt. Simultaneously, he continues to fantasize; visual erotic materials may help.

The stimulation is continued till the man ejaculates, or till 30–60 minutes are over. Some men succeed only on the second or third attempt.

Success rates are 90% for situational anejaculation, 60% for anorgasmic anejaculation and around 50% for neurogenic anejaculation (depending on the level and extent of the spinal lesion).

ELECTROEJACULATION

Electroejaculation involves direct electrical stimulation of the sympathetic nerves innervating the prostate, seminal vesicles, and terminal vas resulting in their contraction and ejaculation.[9]

It is performed using the Seager electroejaculator that delivers an alternating current at an intensity ranging from 0 to 50 V, corresponding to 0 to 1 A of current. The procedure is painful and requires a short general anesthesia unless the patient has spinal cord injury with loss of sensation.

The patient is positioned in the lithotomy or left lateral position and a rectal examination and proctoscopy are performed to rule out any rectal pathology. The electrode is lubricated copiously with jelly and then introduced per rectum with the electrode's stimulation strips facing anteriorly. The electrode is pushed against the prostate and seminal vesicles and the stimulation is started.

The standard technique involves stimulation in one second bursts, starting at 5 V and increasing the stimulus by a couple of volts each time till ejaculation occurs.

If there is no antegrade ejaculation the bladder is catheterized and the urine is checked for retrograde ejaculation.

Electroejaculation is successful in most cases of situational anejaculation and anorgasmic anejaculation and those cases of neurogenic anejaculation where the thoracolumbar outflow is intact. However, the quality of semen is unpredictable and sometimes, inexplicably, count or motility may be poor.[10] Depending on the semen quality, IUI or ICSI can be done with the sample.[11]

SUMMARY

Failure to ejaculate can pose a frustrating problem. Classification of the problem as situational or total, and anorgasmic or orgasmic, provides a practical way of understanding the problem. Diagnosis is easy once the etiological factors are understood. Treatment varies depending on the etiology. The use of vibratory stimulation or electroejaculation is very useful in many of the cases.

REFERENCES

1. Shah R. Management of anejaculation. In: Pandian N (Ed). Handbook of Andrology. Chennai: T.R. Publishers; 1999. pp. 129-39.
2. Wheeler JS Jr, Walter JS, Culkin DJ, et al. Idiopathic anejaculation treated by vibrator stimulation. Fertil Steril. 1988;50:377-79.
3. Hovav Y, Shotland Y, Yaffe H, et al. Electro-ejaculation and assisted fertility in men with psychogenic anejaculation. Fertil Steril. 1996;66:620-23.
4. Soeterik TF, Veenboer PW, Lock TM. Electroejaculation in psychogenic anejaculation. Fertil Steril. 2014;101:1604-8.
5. Kamischke A, Nieschlag E. Treatment of retrograde ejaculation and anejaculation. Hum Reprod Update. 1999;5:448-74.
6. Nehra A, Werner MA, Bastuba M, et al. Vibratory stimulation and rectal probe electroejaculation as therapy for patients with spinal cord injury: semen parameters and pregnancy rates. J Urol. 1996;155:554-9.
7. Chéhensse C, Bahrami S, Denys P, et al. The spinal control of ejaculation revisited: a systematic review and meta-analysis of anejaculation in spinal cord injured patients. Hum Reprod Update. 2013;19:507-26.
8. Hsiao W, Deveci S, Mulhall JP. Outcomes of the management of post-chemotherapy retroperitoneal lymph node dissection-associated anejaculation. BJU Int. 2012;110:1196-200.

9. Bennett C, Seager S, Vasher E, et al. Sexual dysfunction and electroejaculation in men with spinal cord injury: review. BJU. 1991;67:191-4.
10. Meng X, Fan L, Liu J, et al. Fresh semen quality in ejaculates produced by nocturnal emission in men with idiopathic anejaculation. Fertil Steril. 2013;100:1248-52.
11. Ohl DA, Wolf LJ, Menge AC, et al. Electroejaculation and assisted reproductive technologies in the treatment of anejaculatory infertility. Fertil Steril. 2001; 76:1249-55.

CHAPTER
4

Medical Treatment of OATS

PM Gopinath

INTRODUCTION

Approximately 10–15% of all couples of reproductive age groups seek fertility assessment. With an increasing population of working women and the associated delay in the ages of marriage and first child bearing, infertility services are being increasingly utilized.[1] With the advent of assisted reproductive techniques and with the increasing success achieved, the evaluation of the male partner and an attempt at curative treatment is often overlooked. Male factor is involved in about half of the infertility cases. It is essential to identify the pathology and treat the male which may allow couples to improve their fertility potential and conceive through natural intercourse. Figure 4.1 illustrates the various etiology of male factor and its impact on fertility.

The new WHO guidelines on semen analysis[2] is exciting and makes one wonder whether we have over treated the male partners previously. Oligoasthenoteratozoospermia (OATS) known as OAT syndrome is a commonly encountered problem in male infertility.

Treatment options in OATS:

- Medical therapy that may be general or specific
- Surgical therapy
- *Assistance Reprocluctive technology (ART)*: Intrauterine insemination or intracytoplasmic sperm injection

In this article, we are covering only the medical management of OATS.

Specific medical management of OATS is based on identifying reversible causes of infertility and treating them with appropriate medications to achieve a pregnancy. Despite the advancements in diagnostic methodology, no identifiable cause can be found in majority of infertile males. This is referred to as Idiopathic OATS. These patients are treated with nonspecific,

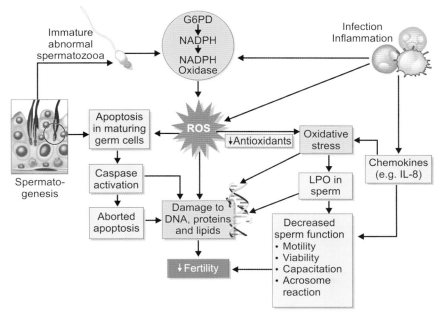

Fig. 4.1: Various etiology of ROS and its impact on fertility.

empirical medications based on theoretical concepts, in an attempt to improve semen parameters and to improve fertility potential.

FACTORS INFLUENCING THE CHOICE OF MEDICAL THERAPY IN OATS

- *Age of the couple and duration of infertility*: A young couple with a short trying time should be given the option of medical therapy in order to buy time to achieve a natural pregnancy. On the other hand, an older couple with a much longer trying time should be counseled to move toward ART.
- *Severity of OATS and realistic chances of improvement expected*: Thus, a patient with severe OATS (<5 million/mL with very poor progressive motility) with no obvious reversible factors is better off being referred for ART.
- *Past illness causing irreversible damage*: For example, a patient who had postmumps orchitis and testicular atrophy, or who was operated for undescended testes. In such patients, it is unlikely that medical therapy will help.
- *Reversible, correctable gonadotoxic factors*? If there is occupational exposure to gonadotoxins (heat, chemical fumes), heavy smoking, recent febrile illness, accessory gland infections, etc., then such patients can be

given supportive medical therapy to buy time for improvement of semen parameters once the gonadotoxic factors are eliminated/modified.

- *Treatment history is imperative*: It is important to know what drugs a patient has already tried in the past (whether they were effective or not) so that there is no repetition. If various drugs have already proved ineffective there is no point in giving further medical therapy.
- Socioeconomic status of the couple should also be considered when deciding medication since many empirical drugs are rather expensive.
- Psychosocial pressures on the couple play an important role in decision making. In a couple that is socially hard pressed for a baby, less time should be spent on medical therapy.

SPECIFIC MEDICAL THERAPY

With history, physical examination, and specific investigations, it is possible to diagnose and treat certain specific medical conditions that will contribute to OATS:

- *Chronic scrotal fungal dermatitis*: This can affect fertility by thickening the scrotal skin and thus increasing the local temperature. This is treated with topical, antifungal plus steroid, creams.
- *Genital tract infection*: The World Health Organization (WHO) defines leukocytospermia as seminal white blood cells (WBC) levels $>1 \times 10^6$/mL (WHO 1999) with the prevalence among male infertility patients being about 10–20%. The clinician must ensure that the laboratory should clearly differentiate between leucocytes and immature germ cells using cytologic staining or immune-histochemical techniques. All men with elevated seminal WBC levels ($>1 \times 10^6$/mL) should be evaluated for a genital tract infection or inflammation, and a semen culture should be performed. Common organisms responsible are *Streptococcus faecalis, Escherichia coli, Chlamydia trachomatis,*[3] and *Ureaplasma urealyticum.* Because of the difficulty of culturing Chlamydia or ureaplasma we often give doxycycline 100 mg/day on an empirical basis for 15 days and then start antibiotics as per culture reports. Commonly used are fluoroquinolones 0.5–1 g/day, cotrimoxazole (sulfamethoxazole 800 mg, trimethoprim 160 mg), or erythromycin 1.5 gm/day. These drugs are administered for 2–3 weeks along with advice of frequent ejaculation. It is also a better option to rotate the antibiotics. However, culture-negative patients with proven leukocytospermia should be treated with anti-inflammatory therapy and frequent ejaculation, because empiric antibiotic therapy generally provides no benefit in these cases and may be harmful. In cases of refractory leukocytospermia, sperm washing can be performed before intrauterine insemination to remove the white cells.

- *Immunologic infertility*: Oral prednisolone is commonly used to suppress antibody production, but no double-blind, randomized large trial has confirmed the efficacy of this therapy. Small studies following different protocols report pregnancy rates between 0% and 44%. Studies in which treatment was continued for >3 months reported a significant increase in the number of pregnancies among those receiving prednisolone compared with placebo.[4]

  Intra Cytoplasmic Sperm Injection (ICSI) is considered to be the treatment of choice for patients with severe sperm autoimmunity. Recently, higher fertilization rates during in vitro fertilization (IVF) were reported in patients with antisperm antibodies who received immunosuppressive therapy compared to IVF without immunosuppressive therapy. Therefore, treatment of antisperm antibodies using corticosteroids should not be prescribed routinely, but can be considered in patients with antisperm antibodies and earlier failed fertilization during IVF or ICSI. High doses of prednisolone should be avoided even on short term due to the rare but catastrophic risk of avascular necrosis of femoral head. It is recommended to use tablet prednisolone 5 mg, thrice-a-day for 10 days, then twice-a-day for 10 days, then once-a-day for 10 days.

- *Chronic epididymo-orchitis*: Many subfertile men have clinical evidence of chronic filarial epididymo-orchitis—residence in an endemic area, enlarged adherent epididymis, thickened cord, lax hydrocoele, h/o hydrocoele surgery, h/o testicular swelling with fever, and occasionally ultrasound evidence of the "filarial dance." Such men sometimes show good improvement in semen parameters after a course of antifilaria therapy (DEC 100 mg thrice-a-day for 20 days in combination with doxycycline 100 mg twice-a-day for 10 days) followed by low-dose steroids as given above.

NONSPECIFIC OR EMPIRICAL THERAPY

In patients with idiopathic OATS, a variety of empirical medical therapies[5] have been recommended. Although there are numerous reports that support a multitude of compounds, the vast majority are nonrandomized studies and unfortunately no medical therapy has demonstrated consistent efficacy in multiple, rigorous, well-controlled, randomized, placebo-controlled trials. Because of isolated case reports and small series demonstrating efficacy of some agents, there is continued hope that they may be effective in select subpopulations of men with idiopathic reproductive dysfunction.

Nonspecific treatments[5] include the following:

- *Hormonal agents*: Androgens, antiestrogens, aromatase inhibitors, gonadotropins
- *Antioxidants*: Glutathione, lycopene, vitamin E

- *Sperm vitalizes*: L-carnitine, coenzyme Q10
- *Nutritional supplements*: Folic acid, zinc, multivitamins, trace elements
- *Miscellaneous*: Indomethacin, Kallikrein, low-dose corticosteroids
- Elimination of gonadotoxic factors.

Hormonal Agents

Androgens

- *Rationale (direct therapy)*: Exogenous androgens, administered at a dose that will not influence the pituitary-gonadal axis, may have a direct stimulatory effect on spermatogenesis or influence sperm transport and maturation through an effect on the epididymis, vas deferens, and seminal vesicles.
- *Drugs used and dosage*: Mesterolone 25 mg thrice daily or testosterone undecanoate[6] 40 mg two to four capsules daily.
- *Rationale (rebound therapy)*: High doses of exogenous androgens will suppress the H-P-T axis and result in azoospermia. Subsequently, after cessation of androgens, the gonadotropin levels will rise again, during which period there may be a rebound increase in sperm counts above baseline. However, rebound therapy has been given up because of uncertain results and risk of permanent azoospermia.

Antiestrogens[7]

- *Rationale*: Antiestrogens inhibit the negative feedback effect of estrogen by blocking estrogen receptors in the hypothalamus, which in turn increases endogenous gonadotropin secretion. In turn, the raised FSH and LH stimulate Sertoli and Leydig cells with a possible improvement in spermatogenesis.
- *Drugs used and dose*: Clomiphene citrate 25 mg daily/alternate days or tamoxifen citrate 10–20 mg daily.

Aromatase Inhibitors

- *Rationale*: Estrogen has a potent negative feedback effect on gonadotropin secretion. Obese men have excessive aromatization, in their fat cells, of testosterone to estrogen resulting in excess estrogen and an altered testosterone to estrogen ratios (T/E). Aromatase inhibitors correct this by inhibiting the peripheral conversion of testosterone and may thereby enhance spermatogenesis.
- *Drugs used and dose*: Letrozole 2.5 mg daily orally, or anastrozole 1 mg daily.

Gonadotropins

- *Rationale*: Some patients with idiopathic infertility may have a subclinical endocrinopathy that results in abnormalities in the bioactivity, half-life, or pulsatility of gonadotropin secretion.[8] Such men may benefit from exogenous gonadotropins despite normal levels on immunoassay.
- *Drugs used*: Human chorionic gonadotropin (1,500 IU i.m three times per week), Human menopausal gonadotropin (37.5–75 IU i.m three times per week).

Antioxidants[9,10]

- *Rationale*: Elevated seminal reactive oxygen species (ROS) levels have been recognized as an independent marker of male factor infertility, irrespective of whether patients have normal or abnormal semen parameters. Spermatozoa are particularly susceptible to oxidative stress-induced damage. Antioxidants in seminal plasma are the most important form of protection available to spermatozoa against ROS. Many studies[9] have supported the use of exogenous antioxidants in the treatment of idiopathic infertility.
- *Drugs used and dose*: Glutathione 250 mg daily (50–600 mg/day), lycopene 4–8 g daily, vitamin E 400–800 mg daily.

Sperm Vitalizers

- *Rationale*: Act through varying mechanisms with a common endpoint of energizing the sperm and making them more capable of fertilization. They may have a role in sperm maturation during the transit through the epididymis. Some of them have an antioxidant action in addition.[5]
- *Drugs used and dose*: L-carnitine and acetyl carnitine 1 g, thrice-a-day; coenzyme Q10 100–300 mg/day.

Nutritional Supplements[9]

- *Rationale*: In our country, majority of the people from the lower socio-economic strata are nutritionally depleted and therefore may not have the necessary levels of vitamins and trace elements to facilitate spermatogenesis.
- *Drugs used*: Multivitamin combinations with zinc, selenium, folic acid, and B12. Various combinations of nutraceuticals are available.[10]

Miscellaneous

- *Rationale*: Some of these therapies have aimed at improving sperm quality by boosting the Kallikrein-Kinin system (kallikreins) or by interfering

with the production of prostaglandins (phosphodiesterase inhibitors, nonsteroidal anti-inflammatory agents)
- *Drugs used*: Kallikreins 600 IU daily; indomethacin.

Elimination of Gonadotoxic Factors

Elimination of chronic exposure to heat at the workplace (furnace, kitchen, etc.) or in leisure activities (sauna, steam bath), cessation of heavy smoking, avoidance of exposure to pesticides (DDT spray) or chemical fumes (aromatic amines), reduction of excessive stress, regularization of diet, and lifestyle can also help some men significantly.

CONCLUSIONS

- As physicians taking care of couples with OATS, it is our duty to give the patients a very clear road map of their course of therapy.
- Therapy must be individualized and it is mandatory that a treatment timeline and endpoints be established prior to initiation of medical therapy.[11]
- When empiric pharmacologic therapy is going to be used, treatment should last at least 3 months to incorporate a full 74-day spermatogenic cycle, and should be followed by a semen analysis.
- If there is significant improvement then the medications should be continued and further improvement monitored monthly. If there is no improvement then the medication should be changed or the therapy may be escalated to ART.
- Patients must be counseled regarding the inconsistent response to medical therapy and to have realistic expectations from the same.
- Most importantly, we must not be guilty of wasting precious time and money over medical therapy when the circumstances call for assisted reproductive therapy.

REFERENCES

1. Petraglia F, Serour GI, Chapron C. The changing prevalence of infertility. Int J Gynecol Obstet. 2013;123(Suppl 2):S4-S8.
2. World Health Organization. WHO Laboratory Manual for the Examination of and Processing of Human Semen, 5th edition. Geneva: World Health Organization; 2010.
3. Cai T, Mazzoli S, Mondaini N, et al. Chlamydia trachomatis infection: challenge for the urologist. Microbiol Res. 2011, vol 2:e14.
4. Hendry WF, Hughes L, Scammell G, et al. Comparison of prednisolone and placebo in subfertile men with antibodies to spermatozoa. Lancet. 1990; 335(8681):85-8.

5. Safarinejad MR, Safarinejad S, Shafiei N, et al. Effects of the reduced form of coenzyme Q10 (ubiquinol) on semen parameters in men with idiopathic infertility: a double-blind, placebo controlled, randomized study. J Urol. 2012; 188(2):526-31.

6. Samplaski MK, Loai Y, Lo K, et al. Testosterone use in the male infertility population: short and longer term effects on semen and hormonal parameters. J Urol. 2013:189(4):E779.

7. Chua ME, Escusa KG, Luna S, et al. Revisiting oestrogen antagonists (clomiphene or tamoxifen) as medical empiric therapy for male infertility: a meta-analysis. Andrology. 2013;1(5):749-57.

8. Nieschlag E, Lenzi A. The conventional management of male infertility. Int J Gynecol Obstet. 2013;123(Suppl 2):S31-5.

9. Showell MG, Brown J, Yazdani A, et al. Antioxidants for male subfertility. Cochrane Database Syst Rev.2011(1):CD007411.

10. Agarwal A, Sekhon LH. Oxidative stress and antioxidants for oligoasthenoteratospermia is it justified? Indian J Urol. 2011;27(1):74-85.

11. Ko EY, Sabanegh ES. The role of over-the-counter supplements for the treatment of male infertility—fact or fiction? J Androl. 2012;33(3):292-308.

CHAPTER
5

Varicocele Surgery: Does It Help?

Vineet Malhotra

INTRODUCTION

It is known that infertility affects 15% of couples of reproductive age. The infertile male has long been an ignored and untreated part of infertility. It has been found that the male factor maybe relevant in up to 50% of all cases of infertility. There has been a lot of interest and controversy regarding the various causes leading to male infertility and their appropriate treatment.[1,2]

Idiopathic infertility is the commonest cause of male factor infertility. Varicoceles (abnormally dilated veins in the pampiniform plexus) are the most common surgically correctable cause of male infertility and are found in 4.4–22.6% of men in the general population. They are present in 20–40% of men with primary infertility and in 75–81% men with secondary infertility.

It was the Greek physician Celsus who, in first century AD, first described varicoceles as swollen and twisted veins over the testicle causing them to be smaller in size. There have been anecdotal reports of crude surgical maneuvers such as wiring of the scrotum to treat these dilated swollen veins.[3-6]

It was much later in the early 1950s that Tulloch reported his results of surgical repair of varicoceles and the resultant improvement in sperm parameters.[7]

There has been immense controversy regarding the standardization of diagnosis and classification of a varicocele. There is also lack of agreement over the need for treatment and the response to treatment.[8]

The predictive value of semen analysis as a marker of male fertility is limited and has been shown by various authors.[9]

Smith et al.[10] reported that up to 25% men with sperm densities below 12.5 million/mL could father a child through spontaneous conception. On the other hand, even with counts of up to 25 million/mL, which is normal by the WHO standards, 10% of men could not father a child with a fertile female.

A more effective outcome parameter would be pregnancy rates since pregnancy is the ultimate endpoint of therapy. When using pregnancy as the endpoint of treatment outcome, it is important to consider the spontaneous pregnancy rate in supposedly infertile couples on no therapy. The spontaneous pregnancy rate is about 1% per month, reaching cumulatively to 26% over 3 years. Obviously, any treatment option being used should improve upon this result. On the other hand, the benefit from an intervention like varicocelectomy may be neutralized by a concomitant untreated female factor.

Good clinical trials require a placebo-controlled, double-blind format. Such a trial, with sham surgery, is ethically impossible in humans. Moreover, randomization on a large scale for such surgeries is also difficult due to the intense social pressure and stress faced by infertile couples resulting in them seeking early intervention. During the course of a multicenter, prospective, randomized trial, in Germany, on radiological embolization of varicoceles, only 67 patients could be randomized in 3 years against a target of 460.[11] Further, follow-up is a major problem among individuals affected by infertility, since they are a young and mobile population. Varicocelectomy results are incremental and pregnancies may occur even 2 years after the surgery. Thus, in another study on surgically treated varicoceles, only 130 out of an original 480 patients remained in the study at the end of 1 year.[12]

There is also inconsistency regarding the populations studied, initial grading of varicocele, age of patient and partner, duration of follow-up, and type of treatment applied. Certain nomograms have been created to predict changes in semen parameters in infertile men after varicocele repair.[13]

Based on current evidence, it is the practice guideline of both the American Urological Association (AUA) and the American Society for Reproductive Medicine (ASRM) that correction of a varicocele should be offered to infertile men with palpable lesions and one or more abnormal semen parameters.[14]

We have attempted to address the issue and provide our view on this debate regarding surgery for varicocele. We will attempt to outline the contentious issues with regards to classification/grading of a varicocele, the effect it may have on fertility, treatment types available, treatment of different grades, unilateral/bilateral varicoceles. We will also discuss the relevance of treating varicoceles with small testicular size, azoospermia, with isolated sperm defects and in adolescents. Finally, we will discuss surgery versus assisted reproductive techniques in the era of Assisted reproductive technology (ART).

DIAGNOSIS AND CLASSIFICATION

Varicoceles are usually diagnosed on clinical examination in an upright position and confirmed by scrotal ultrasound. There is significant examiner bias and variation in classification of varicoceles.[14] The classification of varicoceles on physical examination was described by Dubin[15] (Dubin grading system) into three grades, with grade 3 being visible while the patient is standing, grade 2 is palpable without Valsalva maneuver, and grade 1 is not able to be visualized and only palpable with Valsalva maneuver.

A clinical varicocele is one which is detected on physical examination, either visible or palpable. A nonpalpable enlargement of spermatic veins which is only identifiable by imaging techniques is referred to as a subclinical varicocele.

The imaging techniques used for grading varicoceles include scrotal ultrasound and color Doppler imaging. They have low accuracy and clinical utility as most data have shown a poor correlation between varicoceles detected only on imaging and response to surgery.

For those who utilize scrotal ultrasound as a diagnostic modality, criteria for diagnosing a subclinical varicocele by scrotal ultrasound requires at least the presence of dilated veins with diameter >3.0 mm with concomitant reversal of flow after Valsalva.

Color Doppler Ultrasound Classification of Varicocele (Sarteschi)[16]

Grade Features

- Reflux in vessels in the inguinal channel is detected only during the Valsalva maneuver, while scrotal varicosity is not evident in the standard ultrasound study.
- Small posterior varicosities that extend to the superior pole of the testis. Their diameters increase and venous reflux is seen in the supratesticular region only during the Valsalva maneuver.
- Vessels appear enlarged at the inferior pole of the testis when the patient is evaluated in a standing position; no enlargement is detected if the patient is examined in a supine position. Reflux observed only under during the Valsalva maneuver.
- Vessels appear enlarged even when the patient is studied in a supine position; the dilatation is more marked in the upright position and during the Valsalva maneuver. Testicular hypotrophy is common at this stage.
- Venous ectasia is evident even in the prone decubitus and supine positions. Reflux is observed at rest and does not increase during the Valsalva maneuver.

PATHOPHYSIOLOGY

Varicocele has been postulated to affect testicular function and spermatogenesis through various mechanisms that include elevation of testicular temperature and intratesticular pressure. Other factors such as reflux of toxic metabolites from adrenal glands and hormonal abnormalities have also been implicated. One theory suggests the reduction of blood flow leading to hypoxia and impaired spermatogenesis.

The malfunction of valves of the internal spermatic veins, cremasteric veins, and occasionally the external spermatic veins leads to a reflux and rise of intrascrotal temperatures. This may cause thermal damage to the spermatogenic cells and Leydig cells leading to impaired spermatogenesis.[17-22]

The low sperm concentration is attributed by some researchers to the high germ cell apoptosis usually observed in these men, while the low motility is attributed to the increased concentration of reactive oxygen species.

The exact mechanism by which the above factors contribute to the adverse effect of varicocele on spermatogenesis has not been fully clarified. It is speculated that the main mechanism is DNA damage in sperm heads due to oxidative stress. The latter is caused either by the presence of high levels of reactive oxygen species or by reduced antioxidant capacity. It is interesting to note that these results were confirmed in fertile as well as in infertile men with varicocele. Thus, it becomes obvious that oxidative stress is directly related to varicocele, independent of the fertility status.[23-26]

Nevertheless, oxidative stress is known to have adverse effects on sperm structure and function, such as membrane lipid alterations, disruption of sperm metabolism, reduction of its motility, DNA fragmentation, and reduced overall sperm quality.[27-30]

THE DEBATE

There are several early studies that showed benefit of intervention in cases of subclinical varicoceles. These found results of intervention to be independent of the grade of varicocele and were responsible for the widespread practice of treating all varicoceles by intervention.[31-32] Later, in the early 1990s, studies revealed that there was no significant difference in outcomes between patients with subclinical varicoceles in the observation versus intervention arm.[33-34]

It is now generally agreed that patients with subclinical varicoceles do not warrant any intervention as an isolated causative factor for male infertility.[35]

Several studies have questioned the role of intervention in case of clinical varicoceles and that has been the basis of a Cochrane database review that did not offer conclusive support to intervention [an odds ratio of postoperative spontaneous pregnancy as 1.10 (95% CI: 0.73–1.68)] over expectant management in subfertile couples.[36-40] In a recent meta-analysis published by Kroese et al. the search methodology included the Cochrane Menstrual disorders and Subfertility Group Trials Register (September 12, 2003 to January 2012), the Cochrane Central Register of Controlled trials

(Central) in the Cochrane library issue 1, 2012, Medline (January 1966 to January 2012), Embase (January 1985 to January 2012), PsycINFO (to Week 1, 2012), and reference list of articles.[40b] They have also checked cross-references, references from review articles, and contacted researchers in the field. The meta-analysis included 894 men (10 studies) and showed a combined fixed-effect odds ratio of 1.47 for the outcome of pregnancy (very low quality evidence) favoring intervention.

The study design, patient inclusion criteria, and analysis of these studies have been questioned, as they included patients with normal semen parameters, different methods of intervention, and significant patient dropout.

Madgar et al.[41] studied infertile men with clinical varicoceles and subjected them to intervention versus observation for a period of 12 months. If the patients in the observation group did not report a pregnancy, they were reassigned to the intervention arm. This study revealed a significantly higher pregnancy rate in the immediate (60% in the intervention vs 10% in observation arm) and delayed treatment (44% vs 10%) groups.

The conclusions of Evers and Collins in their systematic review spurred Ficarra et al.[42,43] and Marmar et al.[44] both to re-evaluate the existing data with meta-analyses as well. Ficarra et al. published a meta-analysis including only three of the randomized controlled trials and excluded those where subjects with normal semen analyses or subclinical varicoceles were included. The authors concluded that the heterogeneity of the data and poor quality of study design do not allow for formal analysis. At the same time, the authors used this same argument to refute the conclusions by Evers and Collins. Marmar et al. published a meta-analysis of five studies on surgical repair only on infertile men with clinical varicocele and abnormal semen analysis looking at spontaneous pregnancy rates. The authors included randomized controlled trials and also observational studies. While accepting that this is not standard for the meta-analysis format, the authors state that their inclusion and exclusion criteria allow for less heterogeneity in the population studied and intervention being studied. Odds ratio of spontaneous pregnancy after varicocelectomy was calculated to be 2.87 (95% CI: 1.33–6.20, P = 0.007). Pregnancy rates were also significantly higher in those of treated patients than in not treated (33% vs 15.5%, respectively).

Though varicoceles most commonly present on the left side, this swelling can occur on the right side as well, individually or in unison. *Bilateral* varicocele would seemingly be more detrimental than a unilateral defect. Several investigations have examined whether bilateral repair is similar or superior to one-sided repair. Kondoh et al. reported a small cases series of 27 men with bilateral varicoceles and 40 unilateral left-sided varicoceles and noted less improvements in sperm density in the group with bilateral when compared to the left-sided only group. Four subsequent reports all have demonstrated evidence to support the contrary.[45-47] Scherr et al.[48] prospectively studied 91 men with moderate-to-large left varicocele and small (grade 1) right varicocele and noted significant greater improvements in motile sperm concentrations in those with bilateral repair. Fujisawa et al. and Libman et al. observed significantly greater improvements in concentration and/or motility after bilateral surgical repair.[49,50] Furthermore, Libman et al. and Baazeem et al.[51] noted significantly higher spontaneous pregnancy rates in those with bilateral repair compared to unilateral repair. This evidence would support the notion that subfertility in men with abnormal semen analyses and bilateral palpable varicoceles is the result of an additive effect of both and would justify simultaneous repair, even if small.

Additional studies have examined impact of unilateral or bilateral repair of a clinical varicocele in the presence of a subclinical varicocele with conflicting results. However, grade of varicocele should not dictate treatment. Therefore, in these cases, bilateral repair is likely warranted.

There has been a lot of debate regarding relationship between varicocele and *azoospermia*. Historically, varicocele repair has been as a primary treatment strategy of male infertility with the goal of improving spontaneous pregnancy rates. Severe oligozoospermia and nonobstructive azoospermia are both conditions that significantly reduce a couple's chances at spontaneous pregnancy. Early reports of varicocele repair demonstrate the potential, in some, to induce spermatogenesis and regain the potential for otherwise unassisted fertility. Additionally, the introduction of in vitro fertilization (IVF) and intracytoplasmic sperm injection (ICSI) has allowed for further research on the role of varicocele repair as an adjunct to ART. The presence of varicocele in an azoospermic patient may be causative or coexistent with primary testicular failure and this has led to a disparate management protocol especially with regards to surgical intervention.

It is important to understand the etiology of azoospermia and impaired histology in a patient with clinical varicocele. A small flabby testes with Maturation arrest or Sertoli cell only histology and azoospermia may represent a coexistent pathology or irreversible state and may not benefit from repair of varicocele.

These patients may not show significant benefit even to become candidates for sperm retrieval (TESE) followed by ICSI. Approximately 4–13% of men with a palpable varicocele will present with azoospermia or severe oligoasthenozoospermia. Matthews et al.[52] first published a study looking specifically at this population of men. The authors prospectively evaluated patients after microsurgical varicocelectomy and followed for improvements in semen parameters as well as pregnancies. The majority of the cohort was observed to have return of motile sperm to the ejaculate postoperatively, 55% (12/22) of azoospermic men and 69% (35/51) of those with severe oligoasthenospermia. Mean total motile sperm count increased from $0.08 \pm 0.02 \times 10^6$ to $7.2 \pm 2.3 \times 10^6$ illustrating the potential for men to conceive a subsequent spontaneous pregnancy. Twenty-four (31%) conceived pregnancies, fifteen of which were unassisted. Additionally, testicular atrophy on initial examination had no prognostic value. A subsequent study by Kim et al. noted return of motile sperm as well, but no spontaneous pregnancies.[53]

Varicocele repair led to spermatogenesis and presence of motile sperm in ejaculate of 33% azoospermic men in one study. Fifty-five percent of these men became progressively azoospermic within 1 year of the repair. The study design has been questioned due to lack of a control arm. In another study, 9.6% of men who underwent surgery had sperms which could be used for ICSI.

It is suggested that surgery maybe attempted in azoospermic men with normal-sized testes and large clinical varicoceles though results from different studies has been variable.

Based on the studies by Kim et al., Kadioglu et al., Esteves et al., and Lee et al., those with hypospermatogenesis and maturation arrest at later stages are more likely to see return of motile sperm and pregnancies postoperatively.[54–56]

Pasqualotto et al. and Lee et al. showed that patients are at risk for relapse to azoospermia in the follow-up period and recommend cryopreservation of postoperative samples containing motile sperm.

Pasqualotto et al.[57] reviewed the records of 15 azoospermic men who underwent testicular biopsy and microsurgical varicocelectomy for azoospermia. Forty-seven percent (7/15) men had return of sperm in their ejaculate following surgery with one establishing a spontaneous pregnancy. They noted that even a preoperative biopsy showing germ cell aplasia was not a contraindication to surgery. However, the benefit was not sustained, with five of the seven relapsing to azoospermia after 6 months.

In another retrospective review, Schelegel and Kaufmann reported return of sperm to the ejaculate of 22% of 31 men who underwent microsurgical varicocelectomy.[58] However, only three had adequate motile sperm in the ejaculate for ICSI, while the rest still required testicular sperm extraction (TESE). The authors concluded that such men rarely have adequate sperm in the ejaculate after varicocele repair and most still need TESE. Cakan and Altug reported 13 infertile patients who had complete azoospermia and clinical varicocele, and underwent inguinal varicocele repair. Induction of spermatogenesis was achieved in 3 (23%) patients.[59] None could father a child spontaneously; nor did their sperm result in a successful ICSI. Matthews et al. obtained motile sperm in the semen of 12 out of 22 azoospermic men following varicocele repair; there were three pregnancies (two unassisted and one following ICSI using ejaculated sperm). Only patients whose testicular biopsies showed hypospermatogenesis had motile sperm after surgery. This role of testicular biopsy in nonobstructive azoos-permic men has been reaffirmed in a meta-analysis by Elzanaty.[60]

The role of varicocelectomy in *nonobstructive azoospermia* is unresolved. There are no well-defined predictors of success in this group of patients and while surgery may result in spontaneous conception, this eventuality is rare. Careful case selection (large varicocele, reasonable-sized testes and absence of other causes of infertility) with adequate preoperative counseling is mandatory before considering this option.

The management of children or *adolescents* with varicocele has remained a contentious issue.[61-67]

Current AUA guidelines recommend a conservative, nonsurgical approach for an adolescent with varicocele, as early intervention has not shown to be of any benefit.

The recommendations for early repair of varicoceles in children and adolescents have been listed as follows:
• Varicocele with a significantly small ipsilateral testis
• Additional testicular conditions affecting fertility
• Bilateral palpable varicoceles
• Pathological sperm quality (older adolescents)
• Supranormal response to GnRH stimulation test
• Symptomatic varicocele.

It is AUA best practice policy to follow adolescents annually with testi-cular volume estimation and semen analysis (when possible).

Infertile men with varicoceles have benefitted significantly by the use of *ART* methods to enable them to father children. Varicocele repair has been postulated to downstage and improve the results of ART. Cayan et al.[68] evaluated a cohort of 540 infertile men with clinical varicocele who underwent microsurgical varicocelectomy. The total motile sperm counts were evaluated for each patient preoperatively and postoperatively and the patients were divided into four groups according to the type of assisted reproductive technology for which they qualified: 0–1.5 million, ICSI; 1.5–5 million, IVF; 5–20 million, intrauterine insemination (IUI); 20 million or greater, possibility of spontaneous pregnancy. These men were followed >1 year postoperatively for alterations in semen quality and conception. An overall spontaneous pregnancy rate of 36.6% was achieved after vari-cocelectomy with a mean time to conception of 7 months. Another 31% who preoperatively were assessed as suitable for IVF or ICSI improved enough to become candidates for IUI, while 42% of the IUI candidates gained the potential for spontaneous pregnancy.

Surgery may also help improve the results of assisted reproduction techniques. In a study of 58 patients with a varicocele, patients undergoing varicocelectomy prior to IUI had higher pregnancy rates than those who did not. The authors also noted that while there was no significant improvement in the semen parameters in the two groups, the improved pregnancy rate may be an indicator of improved sperm function, a parameter not evaluated on routine semen analysis.

Marmar et al. initially reported IUI as a possible treatment option for men with history of a varicocele and refractory infertility. Of the 71 couples who underwent 187 inseminations, only 6 achieved a pregnancy. Pregnancy rates were observed to be much higher in a subsequent analysis by Daitch et al. who studied whether varicocele repair improved chance of success with IUI. They studied 58 couples with varicocele-associated infertility, 34 who previously underwent inguinal or subinguinal microsurgical repair and 24 who chose not to undergo repair. Pregnancy rates per cycle were noted to be 6.3% in the untreated group compared to 11.8% in those who underwent surgical repair ($p = 0.04$). Odds of pregnancy were 4.4-fold higher in the surgically treated group favoring varicocelectomy as a strategy to improve chances of pregnancy with assisted means.[69-70]

Several studies have examined effect of varicocele repair on various semen analysis parameters in attempts to correlate varicocelectomy with improved fertility. Unfortunately, these endpoint measurements are limited and more functional endpoint measurements are difficult to assess.

A study by Ashkenazi et al.[71] utilized patients who previously failed to achieve pregnancy following IVF/ICSI, and attempted to attribute subsequent pregnancy success with IVF/ICSI following varicocele repair to the corrective surgery itself. However, it is impossible to attribute this success to the repair procedure and potential improved sperm quality without a more well-controlled study design. Additionally, other studies indicate varicocele repair has no impact on rates of pregnancy following IVF/ICSI, though it may decrease their pursuit of additional ART procedures. Whether this is attributed to improved fertility or simply due to cost, ethical concerns related to ART, or other factors is unknown.[72]

Three cost analyses have been published that both favor varicocele repair as a more cost-effective strategy. Schlegel et al. and Meng et al. reported decision analyses that favor varicocele repair over ART.[73,74] Schlegel estimated cost per live delivery after varicocelectomy and after ICSI to be $26, 268 and $89,091, respectively. However, a subsequent analysis including only men with nonobstructive azoospermia who would require microsurgical TESE favored microTESE as the more cost-effective strategy to varicocelectomy in this subpopulation.[75]

DISCUSSION

The Male Infertility Best Practice Policy Committee of the American Urological Society recommends that varicocele treatment should be offered to the male partner of a couple attempting to conceive when all of the following are present:

- A varicocele is palpable.
- The couple has documented infertility.
- The female has normal fertility or potentially correctable infertility.
- The male partner has one or more abnormal semen parameters or sperm function test results.

In addition, adult men who have a palpable varicocele and abnormal semen analyses findings but are not currently attempting to conceive should also be offered varicocele repair. The indications for repairing varicoceles in adolescents include the presence of significant testicular asymmetry (>20%) demonstrated on serial examinations, testicular pain, and abnormal semen analysis results. Young men with varicoceles but normal ipsilateral testicular volume should be offered follow-up monitoring with annual objective measurements of testicular volume, semen analyses, or both.

Contrary to the opinion offered by the Cochrane Database review, a cost-analysis study by Schlegel showed the significant cost advantage of varicocele repair over ICSI. In addition, varicocele repair had the potential for improving the male factor, rather than using unknown sperm. Intra-cytoplasmic sperm injection also involves IVF, which carries some risk for the female who donates surgically removed eggs.

Cayan et al.[76] specifically evaluated rates of postoperative complications and spontaneous pregnancies and excluded studies involving subclinical varicoceles. After pooling the data from 4,473 men undergoing repair by various techniques, pregnancy rates were compared and significant differences were noted depending on the technique. The highest rates were seen with the microsurgical technique, followed by nonmicrosurgical approaches. This method was also noted to have the least documented recurrences, postoperative hydroceles, or other complications. Agarwal et al. conducted a meta-analysis that included both randomized controlled trials and observational studies in attempts to evaluate the data with more focused attention on men with documented infertility, abnormal semen analysis, and clinical varicoceles. While accepting their study was subject to bias from the variability of semen data in sequential analyses, the authors highlight the significant number of data that document a direct positive relationship between improvements in semen parameters over time and varicocele repair. Agarwal et al. illustrate significant improvements in concentration, motility and morphology in studies evaluating high ligation and microsurgery.[77-78]

CONCLUSIONS

How to treat an infertile male with varicocele is one of the most debated issues in the field of male infertility, specifically with regard to surgical intervention. It is agreed that the surgical repair of varicocele should include a very small group of infertile men. There are no fixed guidelines for selecting the candidates fit for surgery.

Varicoceles are relatively common in the adult male population in general and the infertile male population in particular. In many, but not all, of these infertile men it is can be the cause of their infertility. However, it is important to exercise restraint and clinical judgment before advocating surgery for these patients. Consensus guidelines advocate surgery only for infertile men with clinically obvious varicoceles and persistent seminal abnormalities. About 60% of the operated men will show good improvement in semen parameters. Surgery should also be recommended in adolescent boys with ipsilateral testicular atrophy so as to preserve future fertility. Among the various modes of therapy, microsurgical ligation is the gold standard and should be the procedure of choice. Since success is not guaranteed, and there are no clear predictors of success, it is important to counsel patients about possibility of no benefit after surgery, and discuss the alternative option of assisted reproductive techniques.

Varicocele repair is a reasonable consideration as the primary treatment option when a couple with documented infertility involves a male with a palpable varicocele and suboptimal semen quality and female partner has a normal evaluation. Bilateral repair is warranted when varicoceles are noted on both sides, regardless of grade. However, approach to varicocele treatment should be based on the physician's experience and the additional options available. Assisted reproductive technologies may serve as a viable adjunct or alternative to surgery to improve chances of pregnancy. With improvements in ART laboratory technology, future research efforts are warranted to delineate the benefit of varicocele repair in patients who will require subsequent IVF/ICSI.

Certain additional factors that must be considered before deciding the therapeutic approach of varicocele in infertile couples include:

- The advanced age of the wife (older than 35 years) and high serum FSH levels should drive the decision toward the ICSI solution rather than repair of varicocele.
- In case of chronic presence of varicocele and advanced male age, surgery should be avoided.
- Surgical repair of varicocele is recommended in case of secondary male infertility. On the other hand, if the patient has primary infertility, azoospermia, small testicular size, and high serum FSH levels, the presence of varicocele should be ignored and surgery should be avoided as it indicates a primary testicular failure.
- The diagnosis of Sertoli cell only or early maturation arrest denotes primary testicular failure. Thus, the presence of varicocele should be ignored. On the contrary, the presence of mild or moderate hyposperma-togenesis can be attributed to varicocele in which case surgery can be a reasonable therapeutic approach.

REFERENCES

1. World Health Organisation. The influence of varicocele on parameters of fertility in a large group of men presenting to infertility clinics. Fertil Steril. 1992;57:1289-93.
2. World Health Organisation. Laboratory Manual for the Examination of Human Semen and Sperm–Cervical Mucus Interaction, 4th edition. New York: Cambridge University Press; 1999.
3. Greenberg SH. Varicocele and male infertility. Fertil Steril. 1977;28:699-706.
4. Esteves SC, Miyaoka R, Agarwal A. An update on the clinical assessment of the infertile male. Clinics. 2011;66(4):691-700.
5. Baker HW. Male infertility. Endocrinol Metab Clin North Am. 1994;23:783-93.
6. Saypol DC. Varicocele. J Androl. 1981;2:61.
7. Tulloch WS. Varicocele in subfertility: result of treatment. BMJ. 1955; 4935: 356-8
8. Gorelick JI, Goldstein M. Loss of fertility in men with varicocele. Fertil Steril. 1993;59(3):613–6
9. Mallidis C, Howard EJ, Baker HW. Variation of semen quality in normal men. Int J Androl. 1991;14:99-107.
10. Smith KD, Rodriguez-Rigau LJ, Steinberger E. Relation between indices of semen analysis and pregnancy rate in infertile couples. Fertil Steril. 1977;28:1314-9.
11. Krause W, Muller HH, Schafer H, et al. Does treatment of varicocele improve male fertility? Results of the "Deutsche Varikozelenstudie", a multicentre study of 14 collaborating centres. Andrologia. 2002;34:164-71.
12. Samplaski MK, Yu C, Kattan MW, et al. Nomograms for predicting changes in semen parameters in infertile men after varicocele repair. Fertil Steril. 2014;102(1):68-74.
13. Male Infertility Best Practice Policy Committee of the American Urological Association; Practice Committee of the American Society for Reproductive Medicine. Report on varicocele and infertility. Fertil Steril. 2004;82(Suppl 1): S142-5.
14. Stahl P, Schlegel PN. Standardization and documentation of variccocele evaluation. Curr Opin Urol. 2011;21(6):500-55.
15. Dubin L, Amelar RD. Varicocele size and results of varicocelectomy in selected subfertile men with varicocele. Fertil Steril. 1970;21:606-9.
16. Sarteschi LM. Lo studio del varicocele con eco-Doppler. G Ital Ultrasonologia. 1993;4:43-9.
17. Sharma RK, Agarwal A. Role of reactive oxygen species in male infertility. Urology. 1996;48:835-50.
18. Holland MK, Alvarez JG, Storey BT. Production of superoxide and activity of superoxide dismutase in rabbit epididymal spermatozoa. Biol Reprod. 1982; 27:1109-18.
19. de Lamirande E, Gagnon C. Impact of reactive oxygen species on spermatozoa: a balancing act between beneficial and detrimental effects. Hum Reprod. 1995;10:15-21.
20. Aitken RJ. The Amoroso lecture. The human spermatozoon—a cell in crisis? J Reprod Fertil. 1999;115:1-7.
21. Zini A, de Lamirande E, Gagnon C. Reactive oxygen species in semen of infertile patients: levels of superoxide dismutase- and catalase-like activities in seminal plasma and spermatozoa. Int J Androl. 1993;16:183-8.

22. Allamaneni SS, Agarwal A, Nallella KP, et al. Characterization of oxidative stress status by evaluation of reactive oxygen species levels in whole semen and isolated spermatozoa. Fertil Steril. 2005;83:800-3.

23. Ozdamar AS, Soylu AG, Culha M, et al. Testicular oxidative stress. Effects of experimental varicocele in adolescent rats. Urol Int. 2004;73:343-7.

24. Hendin BN, Kolettis PN, Sharma RK, et al. Varicocele is associated with elevated spermatozoal reactive oxygen species production and diminished seminal plasma antioxidant capacity. J Urol. 1999;161:1831-4.

25. Saleh RA, Agarwal A, Sharma RK, et al. Evaluation of nuclear DNA damage in spermatozoa from infertile men with varicocele. Fertil Steril. 2003;80:1431-6.

26. Mostafa T, Anis TH, El-Nashar A, et al. Varicocelectomy reduces reactive oxygen species levels and increases antioxidant activity of seminal plasma from infertile men with varicocele. Int J Androl. 2001;24:261-5.

27. Cam K, Simsek F, Yuksel M, et al. The role of reactive oxygen species and apoptosis in the pathogenesis of varicocele in a rat model and efficiency of vitamin E treatment. Int J Androl. 2004;27:228-33.

28. Barqawi A, Caruso A, Meacham RB. Experimental varicocele induces testicular germ cell apoptosis in the rat. J Urol. 2004;171:501-3.

29. Onur R, Semercioz A, Orhan I, et al. The effects of melatonin and the antioxidant defence system on apoptosis regulator proteins (Bax and Bcl-2) in experimentally induced varicocele. Urol Res. 2004;32:204-8.

30. Trigo RV, Bergada I, Rey R, et al. Altered serum profile of inhibin B, Pro-alphaC and anti-Mullerian hormone in prepubertal and pubertal boys with varicocele. Clin Endocrinol (Oxf). 2004;60:758-64.

31. Dubin L, Amelar RD. Varicocelectomy: 986 cases in a twelve year study. Urology. 1977;10:446-8.

32. Jarow JP, Ogle SR, Eskew LA. Seminal improvement following repair of ultra-sound detected subclinical varicoceles. J Urol. 1996;155:1287-90.

33. Marsman JW, Schats R. The subclinical varicocele debate. Hum Reprod. 1994;9:1-8.

34. Yamamoto M, Hibi H, Hirata Y, et al. Effect of varicocelectomy on sperm parameters and pregnancy rate in patients with subclinical varicocele: a randomized prospective controlled study. J Urol. 1996;155:1636-8.

35. Unal D, Yeni E, Verit A, et al. Clomiphene citrate versus varicocelectomy in treatment of subclinical varicocele: a prospective randomized study. Int J Urol. 2001;8:227-30.

36. Nieschlag E, Hertle L, Fischedick A, et al. Update on treatment of varicocele: counselling as effective as occlusion of the vena spermatica. Hum Reprod. 1998;13(8):2147-50.

37. Nieschlag E, Hertle L, Fischedick A, et al. Update on treatment of varicocele: counselling as effective as occlusion of the vena spermatica. Hum Reprod. 1998;13:2147-50.

38. Evers JL, Collins JA, Vandekerckhove P. Surgery or embolisation for varicocele in subfertile men. Cochrane Database Syst Rev. 2001;(1):CD000479.

39. Evers JL, Collins JA. Assessment of efficacy of varicocele repair for male sub-fertility: a systematic review. Lancet. 2003;361(9372):1849-52.

40. Evers JL, Collins JA. Surgery or embolisation for varicocele in subfertile men. Cochrane Database Syst Rev. 2004;(3):CD000479.

40b. Kroese AC, de Lange NM, Evers JL, et al. Surgery or embolisation for varicocele in subfertile men. Cochrane Database Syst Rev. 2012;;10:CD000479.

41. Madgar I, Weissenberg R, Lunenfeld B, et al. Controlled trial of high spermatic vein ligation for varicocele in infertile men. Fertil Steril. 1995;63(1):120–4

42. Ficarra V, Cerruto MA, Liguori G, et al. Treatment of varicocele in subfertile men: the Cochrane Review—a contrary opinion. Eur Urol. 2006;49(2):258-63.

43. Ficarra V, Crestani A, Novara G, et al. varicocele repair for infertility: what is the evidence? Eur Urol. 2011;60(4):795-808.

44. Marmar JL, Kim Y. Subinguinal microsurgical varicocelectomy: a technical critique and statistical analysis of semen and pregnancy data. J Urol. 1994; 152:1127-32.

45. Zheng YQ, Gao X, Li ZJ, et al. Efficacy of bilateral and left varicocelectomy in infertile men with left clinical and right subclinical varicoceles: a comparative study. J Urol. 2009;73(6):1236-40.

46. Elbendary MA, Elbadry AM. Right subclinical varicocele: how to manage in infertile patients with clinical left varicocele? Fertil Steril. 2009;92(6):2050-53.

47. Kondoh N, Koh E, Matsui T, et al. Improvement of semen characteristics after surgical repair of bilateral testicular varicocele as compared to unilateral varicocele patients. Arch Androl. 1990;24(1):61-7.

48. Scherr D, Goldstein M. Comparison of bilateral versus unilateral varicocelectomy in men with palpable bilateral varicoceles. J Urol. 1999;162(1):85-8.

49. Fujisawa M, Ishikawa T, Takenaka A. The efficacy of bilateral varicocelectomy in patients with palpable bilateral varicoceles: comparative study with unilateral varicocele. Urol Res. 2003;31(6):407-9.

50. Libman J, Jarvi K, Lo K, et al. Beneficial effect of microsurgical varicocelectomy is superior for men with bilateral versus unilateral repair. J Urol. 2006;176 (6 Pt 1):2602-5.

51. Baazeem A, Boman JM, Libman J, et al. Microsurgical varicocelectomy for infertile men with oligospermia: differential effect of bilateral and unilateral varicocele on pregnancy outcomes. BJU Int. 2009;104(4):524-8.

52. Matthews GJ, Matthews ED, Goldstein M. Induction of spermatogenesis and achievement of pregnancy after microsurgical varicocelectomy in men with azoospermia and severe oligoasthenospermia. Fertil Steril. 1998;70(1):71-5.

53. Kim KH, Lee JY, Kang DH, et al. Impact of surgical varicocele repair on pregnancy rate in subfertile men with clinical varicocele and impaired semen quality: a meta-analysis of randomized clinical trials. Korean J Urol. 2013;54(10):703-9.

54. Kadioglu A, Tefekli A, Cayan S, et al. Microsurgical inguinal varicocele repair in azoospermic men. Urology. 2001;57(2):328-33.

55. Esteves SC, Glina S. Recovery of spermatogenesis after microsurgical subinguinal varicocele repair in azoospermic men based on testicular histology. Int Braz J Urol. 2005;31(6):541-8.

56. Lee JS, Park HJ, Seo JT. What is the indication of varicocelectomy in men with nonobstructive azoospermia? Urology. 2007;69(2):352-5.

57. Pasqualotto FF, Sobreiro BP, Hallak J, et al. Induction of spermatogenesis in azoospermic men after varicocelectomy repair: an update. Fertil Steril. 2006; 85(3):635-9.

58. Schlegel PN, Kaufmann J. Role of varicocelectomy in men with nonobstructive azoospermia. Fertil Steril. 2004;81(6):1585-8.

59. Cakan M, Bakirtas H, Aldemir M, et al. Results of varicocelectomy in patients with isolated teratozoospermia. Urol Int. 2008;80(2):172-6.

60. Elzanaty S. Varicocele repair in non-obstructive azoospermic men: diagnostic value of testicular biopsy—a meta-analysis. Scan J Urol. 2014;8:1-5.

61. Cayan S, Akbay E, Bozlu M, et al. The effect of varicocele repair on testicular volume in children and adolescents with varicocele. J Urol. 2002;168:731-4.

62. Thomas JC, Elder JS. Testicular growth arrest and adolescent varicocele: does varicocele size make a difference? J Urol. 2002;168:1689-91.

63. Lund L, Tang YC, Roebuck D, et al. Testicular catch-up growth after varicocele correction in adolescents. Pediatr Surg Int. 1999;15:234-7.

64. Rivilla F, Casillas JG. Testicular size following embolization therapy for paediatric left varicocele. Scand J Urol Nephrol. 1997;31:63-5.

65. Haddad NG, Houk CP, Lee PA. varicocele: a dilemma in adolescent males. Pediatr Endocrinol Rev. 2014;11(Suppl 2):274-83.

66. Pinto KJ, Kroovand RL, Jarow JP. Varicocele related testicular atrophy and its predictive effect upon fertility. J Urol. 1994;152:788-90.

67. Ku JH, Son H, Kwak C, et al. Impact of varicocele on testicular volume in young men: significance of compensatory hypertrophy of contralateral testis. J Urol. 2002;168:1541-4.

68. Cayan S, Shavakhabov S, Kadio lu A. Treatment of palpable varicocele in infertile men: a meta-analysis to define the best technique. J Androl. 2009;30(1):33-40.

69. Marmar JL, Agarwal A, Prabakaran S, et al. Reassessing the value of varicocelectomy as a treatment for male subfertility with a new meta-analysis. Fertil Steril. 2007;88(3):639-48.

70. Daitch JA, Bedaiwy MA, Pasqualotto EB, et al. Varicocelectomy improves intrauterine insemination success rates in men with varicocele. J Urol. 2001;165(5):1510-13.

71. Ashkenazi J, Dicker D, Feldberg D, et al. The impact of spermatic vein ligation on the male factor in in vitro fertilization-embryo transfer and its relation to testosterone levels before and after operation. Fertil Steril. 1989;51(3):471-4.

72. Evers JH, Collins J, Clarke J. Surgery or embolisation for varicocele in subfertile men. Cochrane Database Syst Rev. 2009;(1):CD000479.

73. Schlegel P. Is assisted reproduction the optimal treatment for varicocele-associated male infertility? A cost effective analysis. Urology. 1997;49(1):83-90.

74. Meng MV, Greene KL, Turek PJ. Surgery or assisted reproduction? A decision analysis of treatment costs in male infertility. J Urol. 2005;174(5):1926-31.

75. Lee R, Li PS, Goldstein M, et al. A decision analysis of treatments for nonobstructive azoospermia associated with varicocele. Fertil Steril. 2009;92(1):188-96.

76. Cayan S, Erdemir F, Ozbey I, et al. Can varicocelectomy significantly change the way couples use assisted reproductive technologies? J Urol. 2002;167(4):1749-52.

77. Gabriele R, Conte M, Egidi F, et al. Results of surgical treatment of varicocele in male infertility. Curr Opin Urol. 2012;22(6):489-94.

78. Agarwal A, Deepinder F, Cocuzza M, et al. Efficacy of varicocelectomy in improving semen parameters: new meta-analytical approach. Urology. 2007;70(3):532-8.

CHAPTER

6

Evaluation and Management of Azoospermia

Carlos Balmori

DEFINITION, DIAGNOSIS, AND EPIDEMIOLOGY

Azoospermia is defined as the complete absence of sperm in the ejaculation. The presence of even a small number of spermatozoa is defined as cryptozoospermia. Aspermia is distinct from azoospermia and is defined by the complete absence of seminal fluid emission at time of orgasm.

The diagnosis must be confirmed by centrifugation of a semen specimen at 3,000 g for 15 minutes at room temperature with a high-powered microscopic examination of the pellet. The presence of any mature sperm in the semen excludes the possibility of complete absence of spermatogenesis.

The semen analysis should be performed according to the 2010 World Health Organization guidelines, and at least two semen samples obtained > 2 weeks apart should be examined.[1] Azoospermia is found in approximately 1% of all men and 10–15% of infertile males.[2]

ETIOLOGICAL CLASSIFICATION

Traditionally azoospermia is classified into obstructive azoospermia (OA) and *nonobstructive* azoospermia (NOA).[3] In obstructive cases spermatogenesis is normal but there is obstruction in the seminal ducts, while in nonobstructive cases there is deficient, or absent spermatogenesis. Obstructive azoospermia and nonobstructive azoospermia can be further divided into congenital, acquired, or iatrogenic according to their etiology (Table 6.1). Azoospermia due to ejaculatory duct dysfunction and hypogonadotrophism are rare, accounting for about 2% of azoospermia.[4]

Another clinical classification[5] is *pretesticular* (due to deficient hormonal stimulation of the testis), *testicular* (due to testicular dysfunction), and *post-testicular* (due to seminal ductal obstruction or dysfunction) (Table 6.2). Whereas the pretesticular and post-testicular causes of azoospermia frequently are correctable, the testicular causes of azoospermia are not.

Table 6.1: Etiology of OA and NOA.		
	Type of azoospermia	
Etiology	Obstructive azoospermia (OA)	Nonobstructive azoospermia (NOA)
Congenital	• Congenital bilateral absence of the vas deferens (CBAVD) • Young syndrome • Prostatic cysts (Müllerian cysts) • Idiopathic epididymal obstruction	• Cryptorchidism • Sertoli only syndrome • Steiner's syndrome • Reifenstein's syndrome • Kallmann's syndrome • Noonan syndrome • Klinefelter's syndrome • Prader-Willy's syndrome • Y-chromosome microdeletions • Androgen insensitivity syndrome • Meiotic and meiosis abnormalities during spermatogenesis
Acquired	• Vasectomy • Prostatitis, epididymitis • Testicular trauma	• Orchitis • Testicular neoplasm • Testicular injury (trauma, torsion) • Pituitary tumor • Varicocele
Iatrogenic	• Postsurgical (hernia, scrotum)	• Radiation • Medication (cytotoxic, antiandrogens, cimetidine, ketoconazole, spironolactone, testosterone) • Postsurgical (bladder neck, retroperitoneal)

EVALUATION OF AZOOSPERMIC PATIENTS

Aims

- To determinate the cause and any treatment options that may be effective.
- To recognize that azoospermia may be the initial manifestation of a severe medical condition.
- To estimate the probability of recovering sperm in patients with NOA.
- To assess the risks of genetic abnormalities in these males.

Clinical Assessment

The initial evaluation of the azoospermic male patient should be rapid, noninvasive, and cost-effective. A great number of conditions causing azoospermia in men can be diagnosed by history, physical examination,

Table 6.2: Classification of azoospermia based upon the area problem.

Area Problem	Etiology	
Pretesticular	Hypogonadotrophic hypogonadism	• Idiopathic • Kallmann's syndrome • Pituitary tumors
Testicular	• Idiopathic • Cryptorchidism • Cytotoxic therapy • Irradiation • Testicular neoplasm • Systemic illness (Cirrhosis, renal failure) • Viral or inflammatory orchitis • Drugs • Vascular injury • Varicocele • Testicular torsion • Genetic disorders • Y-chromosome microdeletions	
Post-testicular	Seminal ducts obstruction	• Vasectomy • Postsurgical (hernia, scrotum) • Postinfective (epididymitis, orchitis, prostatitis) • Congenital bilateral absence of the vas deferens (CBAVD) • Idiopathic epididymal obstruction • Prostatic cysts (Müllerian cysts) • Young's syndrome
	Ejaculatory ducts dysfunction	• Retrograde ejaculation • Anejaculation • Spinal cord injury • Neurological illness • Diabetes mellitus • Erectile dysfunction • Postsurgery (retroperitoneal lymphadenectomy, bladder neck)

semen analysis, and hormonal and genetic tests. Further evaluation can then be done as necessary. A rational approach is necessary to perform the appropriate workup and to choose the best treatment options for the couple.

History

A detailed history must include information about not only medical and surgical problems, but also developmental issues, occupational and social habits, and exposures.

- *Childhood illnesses*: This includes questions related to cryptorchidism, mumps, hypospadias, gynecomastia, herniorrhaphy or scrotal surgery, and the onset of pubertal changes. Precocious or delayed puberty may be the sign of a serious underlying endocrinologic disorder. Hormonally active tumors from the testicle, adrenal gland, or pituitary, along with adrenal hyperplasia, primary testicular insufficiency, or end-organ androgen insensitivity, may alter the onset of puberty. Testicular torsion and trauma may result in testicular atrophy and the production of antisperm antibodies.

- *Adult illnesses*: A history of anosmia in combination with azoospermia or severe oligospermia and low gonadotropins suggests Kallmann's syndrome. Bronchiectasis, sinusitis, and OA can be observed in Young's syndrome or cystic fibrosis. Smallpox, postpubertal mumps, prostatitis, orchitis, seminal vesiculitis, and urethritis may lead to azoospermia. Liver and renal diseases lead to hypogonadism and feminization because of primary testicular failure and increased estrogen levels. Obesity causes an increased peripheral conversion of testosterone to estrogen and decreased LH pulse amplitude. Ejaculatory dysfunction may be secondary to diabetes mellitus. Patients should be questioned about recent fevers and systemic illness, because spermatogenesis may be adversely affected for 2–3 months, and semen analysis must be repeated at timely intervals up to 6 months after such episodes. Spinal cord injury can cause infertility through epididymal, testicular, prostatic, seminal vesicular, or ejaculatory dysfunction.

- *Medical or surgical treatments*: Many therapeutic drugs are associated with decreased sperm production and sperm quality: anabolic steroids, Dilantin, manganese, colchicine, methadone, methotrexate, phenytoin, Thioridazine, calcium channel blockers, spironolactone, cyproterone, ketoconazole, cimetidine, tetracycline, nitrofurantoin, valproic acid, or sulfasalazine. History of cancer and related chemotherapy or radiation must be sought, not only for the potential effects on spermatogenesis, but also for determination of a time interval after which retrieved sperm can be safely used after such therapies.

- *Sexual history*: Anejaculation may masquerade as azoospermia when the man collects urethral secretions or urine in lieu of semen.

- *Environmental or occupational assaults*: Overexposure to these assaults can cause azoospermia, either by direct suppression of sperm production or by affecting hormone secretion. Some chemicals that affect sperm production are as follows: free oxygen radicals, pesticidal chemicals (DDT, aldrin, dieldrin, PCPs, dioxins, and furans) with estrogen-like effects, plastic softening chemical like phthalates, and hydrocarbons (ethylbenzene, benzene, toluene, and xylene). Chronic exposure to heavy metals such as lead, cadmium, or arsenic may affect the hypothalamic-pituitary axis and cause azoospermia in otherwise healthy men.

- *Social habits and exposures*: Emotional stress or excessive heat exposure may cause a temporary decrease in sperm production but rarely azoospermia. The same applies to tobacco and alcohol. The relationship of tobacco with sperm concentration is shown in several studies.[6] Meanwhile, it seems to be difficult to relate alcohol consumption with an impairment of sperm counts as a single factor.[7]

Physical Examination

Signs of endocrinopathy or genetic alterations as a cause of azoospermia should be sought. The amount and distribution of body hair, including beard growth, axillary hair, and pubic hair should be noted. The ethnic origin of the patient should be considered in this assessment. Any decrease in body hair or decrease in beard growth should also be noted. The presence and degree of gynecomastia should be recorded. The presence of galactorrhea would suggest pronounced hyperprolactinemia, usually associated with some degree of hyperestrogenism.[8] Eunuchoid stature, subvirilization, and disproportionately long extremities can be associated with genetic disorders such as Klinefelter's syndrome (KS) characterized by testosterone deficiency.[9]

The genital examination should include palpation of the spermatic cord, the aspect and symmetry of the scrotum, and testicular mobility and consistency. Length and width of the testes, or its volume, should be measured by using calipers, a Prader orchidometer, or ultrasound. Some testicular disorders may selectively affect production of sperm without influencing production of testosterone. Because approximately 85% of testicular mass consists of germinal tissue, a reduced germinal cell mass would be associated with a reduced testicular size and a soft consistency.

Testicular consistency should be noted. If the germinal epithelium was damaged before puberty, the testes are generally small and firm. If postpubertal damage occurred, the testes are usually small and soft.

A through palpation of the epididymis—its caput, corpus, and cauda—is of importance. Epididymal enlargement, induration, and cysts are indicative of OA.

The presence of the vas deferens should be ascertained while palpating the spermatic cord. The complete absence bilaterally of the vasa is observed in men with mutations in one or both copies of the *CF* gene. Sometimes these men may have only a partial defect in the vas. Surgical scars in the inguinal or scrotal area may indicate possible injuries to the testicular blood supply and/or vas deferens.

Abnormal shapes of the penis or wrong opening of the urethral meatus are not a cause of azoospermia.

A complete physical examination of males with azoospermia must include a rectal examination to exclude ejaculatory duct obstruction. Midline prostatic cysts, such as Müllerian duct cysts, and dilated seminal vesicles can be palpated; a definite diagnosis can be confirmed by transrectal ultrasound scanning and deferentovesiculography.[10] Prostatic induration or tenderness supports a diagnosis of prostatitis.

One study has investigated whether anogenital distance (AGD) could distinguish men with OA from those with NOA. Anogenital distance is a marker for endocrine disruption in animal studies in which decreased male AGD has been associated with testicular dysfunction.[11]

Semen Analysis

Once azoospermia has been established, semen analysis can provide additional valuable information about the likely origin of azoospermia. It allows assessment of accessory glands' function, and detection of immunological, inflammatory, or infectious problems.

A low ejaculate volume indicates absence of seminal vesicular fluid. This is commonly due to absence of the seminal vesicles in association with vas aplasia, but may also occur if there is ejaculatory duct obstruction. Occasionally, this may be due to incomplete ejaculation or partial retrograde ejaculation, or severe hypogonadism resulting in failure of accessory gland secretions. Large volumes are sometimes found in association with infection of the genital tract or after long periods of sexual abstinence.

The pH is determined by acidic secretions of the prostate and alkaline secretions of the seminal vesicles. If the pH exceeds 8.0, infection should be suspected with decreased secretion of acidic products by the prostate, such as citric acid. Abnormal pH may also be recorded in cases of incomplete ejaculation. Acidic pH (<6.5) is found in cases of agenesis or obstruction of the seminal vesicles.

The presence of agglutination is suggestive of, but not sufficient evidence to prove, the existence of an immunological factor.[12]

The biochemical analysis of semen enables us to detect disturbances for each organ involved in seminal fluid production. The fructose level for seminal vesicular function, citrate or acid phosphatase for the prostate gland, and free carnitine as an index of epididymal function.[13]

Hormonal Analysis

According to AUA Infertility Best Practice Statement,[14] the minimum initial hormonal evaluation should consist of measurements of serum follicle-stimulating hormone (FSH) and serum testosterone levels. If the testosterone level is low, a repeat measurement of total and free testosterone (or bioavailable testosterone) as well as determination of serum luteinizing hormone (LH) and prolactin (PRL) levels should be obtained.

LH and FSH are synthesized in the pituitary gland, released into the systemic blood circulation, and carried to the target end organs—the gonads. The pituitary also secretes PRL. In the testis, LH stimulates testosterone secretion and FSH is important in the initiation and maintenance of spermatogenesis. The secreted testicular androgens—testosterone and its activated form dihydrotestosterone (DHT)—act on numerous target end organs causing the development of male secondary sexual characteristics and inhibiting the pituitary secretion of LH and FSH. Spermatogenesis is dependent on pituitary FSH and on intratesticular testosterone. FSH and androgens seem to have different preferential sites of action during spermatogenesis.

In the presence of normal spermatogenesis, FSH secretion is regulated by negative inhibition from inhibin. With primary testicular failure, inadequate Leydig and Sertoli cell functions result in elevated gonadotropin levels with normal or low testosterone levels. Hypothalamic or pituitary dysfunction resulting in inadequate levels of gonadotropins causes low peripheral levels of testosterone and an absence of spermatogenesis. Men who have selective injury to the germinal epithelium (seminiferous tubules) have elevated serum FSH, but normal LH and testosterone levels. In OA, FSH levels are normal, but normal levels do not exclude a testicular cause of azoospermia—FSH is normal in 40% of men with primary spermatogenic failure. Inhibin B seems to have a higher predictive value for normal spermatogenesis[15] (Table 6.3).

Elevated FSH levels have been associated with a low probability for the retrieval of spermatozoa in men and lower pregnancy rates in their female partners using random biopsy testicular sperm extraction (TESE) techniques. Although FSH reflects the predominant pattern of spermatogenesis, it may not reflect isolated areas of spermatogenesis within the testis. Thus, micro-TESE has been shown to be more successful in sperm retrieval than a single biopsy or multiple random biopsies.[16]

Genetic Analysis

Genetic factors explain 21–29% of azoospermia, and another 12–41% of azoospermic cases are idiopathic and most likely related to unknown

Table 6.3: Hormonal status and clinical diagnosis of azoospermia.

Clinical Status	FSH	Inhibin B	LH	Testosterone
• Normal	Normal	Normal	Normal	Normal
• Spermatogenic arrest	Normal	Normal	Normal	Normal
• Aplasia germinal	High	Low	Normal	Normal
• Hypergonadotropic hypogonadism (testicular failure)	High	Low	High	Normal or Low
• Hypogonadotropic hypogonadism	Low		Low	Low

genetic factors.[17] Some researchers believe that approximately 75% or more cases of infertility have a genetic basis, but our current ability to diagnose these defects remains limited.[2] A particular difficulty is the huge number of candidate genes to be studied; there are >2,300 genes expressed in the testis alone, and hundreds of those genes influence reproductive function in humans and could contribute to male infertility.

Cytogenetic analysis of patients with azoospermia and severe oligozoospermia is mandatory before infertility treatment with assisted reproduction technologies. We must research the main genetic factors related to azoospermia: chromosomal abnormalities, cystic fibrosis gene mutations, and Y-chromosome microdeletions.

Chromosomal abnormalities can be identified by karyotype of peripheral leukocytes in approximately 7% of infertile men. The prevalence of such abnormalities relates inversely to the sperm concentration,[18] being 10–15% in azoospermic men, 5–12.8% in oligospermic men, and <1–1.1% in patients with normozoospermia.[19-20] The most common chromosomal aberrations that are associated with severe spermatogenic defects are sex chromosome aneuploidies and chromosomal translocations. Among the various cytogenetic abnormalities, KS is the major cytogenetic/sex chromosome/numerical anomaly that is detected in infertile men.[17]

Klinefelter's syndrome is the most prevalent chromosomal disorder in humans, with an estimated frequency of 1:500 to 1:1,000 men.[21] It is also the most frequent genetic cause of azoospermia.[22] Men with KS have an extra paternal X chromosome in nearly half of all cases. In nonmosaic KS of both paternal and maternal origin, the extra X chromosome is the result of meiotic nondisjunction or possibly of premature separation of sister chromatids.[23-24]

Approximately 8% of adult men with KS have sperm present, with sperm concentrations $<1 \times 10^6$/mL, and impairment in sperm motility and morphology.[25] In those patients with azoospermia and Sertoli cell-only pattern on pretreatment testicular histology, sperm retrieval using microdissection TESE was successful in 70% of the cases.[26] Given the potential for increased chromosomal abnormalities in the offspring of men with KS, preimplantation genetic diagnosis of embryos obtained using TESE-ICSI has been recommended.[27]

Patients with congenital bilateral absence of vas deferens (CBAVD) or unexplained OA and low-semen volume should be tested for abnormalities of the cystic fibrosis transmembrane conductance regulator *(CFTR)* gene. The *CFTR* gene is located on chromosome 7 q31.2 and has been implicated in the formation of excurrent seminal ducts.[28] Patients with congenital bilateral absence of vas deferens accounts for ~1–2% of the population of infertile, but otherwise healthy, males and up to 25% of those with OA. Imaging studies and surgical exploration generally are unnecessary for diagnosis but may help to identify other abnormalities associated with vasal agenesis. Patients with congenital bilateral absence of vas deferens males, having detectable CFTR mutations in most of them, are able to father their children with help of assisted reproductive technologies, so CFTR mutations may be artificially transmitted to the offspring as a consequence. Therefore, genetic testing should be offered to these CBAVD patients before undergoing assisted reproduction, which allows for better evaluation of the genetic risk for the offspring.[29] Many mutations of the CFTR are undetectable using commercial kits and hence it should be assumed that the male is a carrier, even when testing negative, and testing should be offered to his female partner to exclude the possibility that she too may be a carrier.[19]

Yq microdeletion is another recognized cause of spermatogenic failure, causing azoospermia or severe oligozoospermia. Yq microdeletions involve loss of one or more of three discreet loci on the q arm of Y chromosome.[30]

The prevalence of Yq microdeletions is ~7.4%. In an azoospermic population, the prevalence is higher (9.7%), while in oligozoospermic men, the prevalence is 6.0%. The Yq contains three "azoospermia factor (AZF)" regions: AZFa, AZFb, and AZFc. Deletions of the complete AZFc region are most frequently detected (69%), followed by deletions of the AZFb region (14%) and deletions of the AZFa region (6%).[31] Yq microdeletions contribute only marginally to the totality of human male infertility, but when present, the use of ICSI may allow for the transmission of such mutations to the next generation. Couples should be offered this information, as they must understand that their male offspring will almost certainly be subfertile and require reproductive care.[32]

The occurrence and type of microdeletion correlates with testicular phenotype and is a good predictor of sperm retrieval during microdissection TESE. Sperm retrieval is not successful in those patients with AZFa, AZFb, AZFb+c, and complete Yq deletions; however, patients with AZFc have better prognosis, and sperm retrieval is possible.[33] Also, oligozoospermic men with microdeletions have been reported to progress to azoospermia over time, and higher incidence of poor-quality embryos has been observed in couples where the male partner has microdeletions.[34]

TREATMENT OF AZOOSPERMIA

Some men can be managed with surgical or medical treatment. In other cases, operative spermatic recovery techniques will be necessary.

Medical Management

Less than 3% of NOA men have a primary hormonal etiology[35] like hypogonadotropic hypogonadism.

Among men with NOA, gonadotropin therapy for hypogonadotropic hypogonadism is the only specific indication that has universally shown an improvement in semen analysis and pregnancy rates. Gonadotropins (hCG and rFSH in combination) are the standard therapy, while GnRH therapy is reserved for nonresponders. Avoiding the use of drugs that inhibit the hypothalamic axis, such as tranquilizers or steroids can be useful in some cases. The medical management of other forms of NOA, such as patients who have primary Leydig cell damage, remains empirical. Drug therapy with aromatase inhibitors and gonadotropins shows potential promise in improving outcomes in men requiring surgical sperm retrieval, but there is lack of level I clinical evidence for this indication.[36]

Surgical Management

Microsurgical reconstruction may be possible when OA has resulted from previous vasectomy, or epididymal obstruction. The main surgical techniques are the vasovasostomy and the vasoepididymostomy. Occasionally, transurethral resection of obstructed ejaculatory ducts can be curative. Some men with large varicoceles may have reappearance of sperm in the ejaculate after varicocelectomy.

Vasovasostomy

About 2–6% men who undergo vasectomy will desire reversal of their vasectomy at a later time.[37] Vasectomy reversal can be performed in a variety of ways. Variability exists in the size and number of sutures used as well as in the number of layers anastomosed. Microsurgical vasovasostomy, as described by Owen[38] and Silber,[39] is the gold standard with overall patency and pregnancy rates reported by the vasovasostomy Study Group of 86% and 52%, respectively.[40] While a two-layer technique has been advocated, it is often tedious and time-consuming, and no difference has been demonstrated compared to a microsurgical one-layer closure. Fibrin glue vasovasostomy is potentially less time-consuming than standard microsurgical vasovasostomy.[41]

Vasoepididymostomy

The need to perform vasoepididymostomy has been reported to be as high as 62% in patients undergoing reversal 15 or more years after vasectomy.[42] Patients with epididymal obstruction from other causes (congenital or infection) are also candidates for vasoepididymostomy. Nonmicrosurgical epididymovasostomy, based upon the creation of a fistula between several openings in the epididymal tubule and the lumen of the vas, was first described by Martin.[43] Dubin and Amelar[44] suggested the use of loupes.

Later microsurgical techniques were developed. End-to-end and end-to-side anastomoses (Schlegel and Goldstein[45]) and longitudinal and triangulation intussusception (Schiff[46]) are currently favored techniques. With epididymovasostomy restoration of patency can be achieved in 65% of cases with a 38% natural pregnancy rate.[47]

In men undergoing vasostomy or vasoepididymostomy, sperm retrieval and cryopreservation during the operation is recommended for surgical and pregnancy failure.[48]

SPERM RETRIEVAL TECHNIQUES

Unreconstructable OA and NOA have historically been relatively untreatable conditions that required the use of donor spermatozoa. ICSI has transformed treatment for this type of severe male factor infertility. Sperm retrieval with IVF/ICSI is also preferred to surgical treatment when the female partner is advanced in age or there is female infertility requiring IVF. Depending on the type of azoospermia, sperm can be retrieved either from the epididymis or the testes.

The sperm retrieval methods can be either open surgery or percutaneous acquisition. Both of them can be performed by macro- or microsurgical techniques (Table 6.4; Figs. 6.1A to C). Historical prognostic factors for sperm recovery in NOA are related to the clinical, laboratory, and surgical technique, the testicular tissue processing method in the gamete laboratory; and the histological pattern of the testis. Nonobstructive azoospermia remains the most challenging diagnosis for andrologists, and there are no positive prognostic factors that guarantee sperm recovery for these patients. The only reliably negative prognostic factor is the presence of AZFa and AZFb microdeletions.[49]

Table 6.4: Sperm retrieval techniques.

Type of surgery	Open surgery	Percutaneous acquisition
Nonmicrosurgical	• Open epididymal fine—needle aspiration	• Percutaneous epididymal sperm aspiration (PESA)
	• Testicular sperm extraction (TESE)	• Percutaneous testicular sperm aspiration (TESA)
	• Single seminiferous tubule biopsy	• Percutaneous testicular fine-needle aspiration (TEFNA)
Microsurgical	• Microsurgical epididymal sperm aspiration (MESA)	
	• Microsurgical testicular sperm extraction (Micro-TESE)	

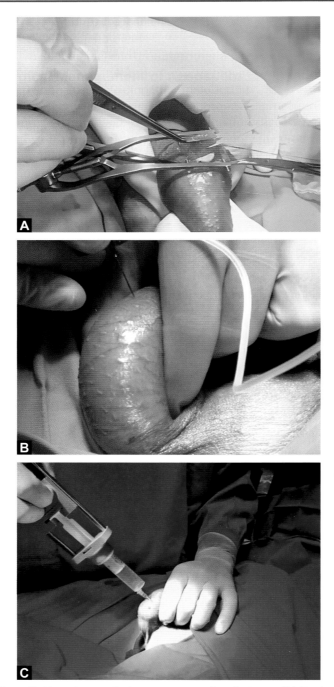

Figs. 6.1A to C: Nonmicrosurgical sperm retrieval techniques. (A) Testicular sperm extraction (TESE). (B) Percutaneous epididymal sperm aspiration (PESA). (C) Percutaneous testicular sperm aspiration (TESA).

REFERENCES

1. WHO. WHO Laboratory Manual for the Examination and Processing of Human Semen, 5th edition. Geneva: WHO Press; 2010.
2. Cocuzza M, Alvarenga C, Pagani R. The epidemiology and etiology of azoospermia. Clinics. 2013;68(S1):15-26.
3. Ezeh UI. Beyond the clinical classification of azoospermia. Hum Reprod. 2000;15(11): 2356-9.
4. Hull MGR, Glazener CMA, Kelly NJ, et al. Population study of causes, treatment and outcome of infertility. Brit Med J. 1985;291:1693-7.
5. Sharif K. Reclassification of azoospermia: the time has come? Hum Reprod. 2000;15(2): 237-8.
6. Ramlau-Hansen C, Thulstrup AM, Aggerholm AS, et al. Is smoking a risk factor for decreased semen quality? A cross-sectional analysis. Hum Reprod. 2007;22:188-96.
7. Martini AC, Molina RI, Estofán D, et al. Effects of alcohol and cigarette consumption on human seminal quality. Fertil Steril. 2004;82:374-7.
8. Petak SM. AACE Hypogonadism Guidelines. Endocr Pract. 2002;8(6):440-56.
9. Gudeloglu A, Parekattil SJ. Update in the evaluation of the azoospermic male. Clinics. 2013;68(S1):27-34.
10. Shebel HM, Farg HM, Kolokythas O, et al. Cysts of the lower male genitourinary tract: embryologic and anatomic considerations and differential diagnosis. Radiographics. 2013;33(4):1125-43.
11. Eisenberg ML, Shy M, Walters RC, et al. The relationship between anogenital distance and azoospermia in adult men. Int J Androl. 2012;35(5):726-30.
12. Hoover P, Naz RK. Do men with prostate abnormalities (prostatitis/benign prostatic hyperplasia/prostate cancer) develop immunity to spermatozoa or seminal plasma? Int J Androl. 2012;35(4):608-15.
13. Wetterauer U. Recommended biochemical parameters for routine semen analysis. Urol Res. 1986;14(5):241-6.
14. Jarow J, Sigman M, Kolettis PN, et al. 2010. The evaluation of the azoospermic male: AUA best practice statement, reviewed and revised 2011. American Urological Association Education and Research, Inc. http://www.auanet.org/common/pdf/education/clinical-guidance/Male-Infertility-b.pdf.Accessed Feb.2014
15. Jungwirth A, Giwercman A, Toumaye H, et al. European Association of Urology Guidelines on Male Infertility: The 2012 Update. Eur Urol. 2012;62(2):324-32.
16. Ramasamy R, Lin K, Gosden LV, et al. High serum FSH levels in men with nonobstructive azoospermia does not affect success of microdissection testicular sperm extraction. Fertil Steril. 2009;92(2):590-93.
17. Hamada AJ, Esteves SC, Agarwal A. A comprehensive review of genetics and genetic testing in azoospermia. Clinics. 2013;68(S1):39-60.
18. Clementini E, Palka C, Iezzi I, et al. Prevalence of chromosomal abnormalities in 2078 infertile couples referred for assisted reproductive techniques. Hum Reprod. 2005;20:437-42.
19. ASRM Practice Committee. Evaluation of the azoospermic male. Fertil Steril. 2008;90:S74-7.
20. Pylyp LY, Spinenko LO, Verhoglyad NV, et al. Chromosomal abnormalities in patients with oligozoospermia and non-obstructive azoospermia. J Assist Reprod Genet. 2013;30:729-32.

21. Bojesen A, Juul S, Gravholt CH. Prenatal and postnatal prevalence of Klinefelter syndrome: a national registry study. J Clin Endocrinol Metab. 2003;88:622-6.

22. Tuttelmann F, Werny F, Cooper TG, et al. Clinical experience with azoospermia: aetiology and chances for spermatozoa detection upon biopsy. Int J Androl. 2011;34:291-8.

23. Hassold T, Hunt P. To err (meiotically) is human: the genesis of human aneuploidy. Nat Rev Genet. 2001;2:280-91.

24. Thomas NS, Hassold TJ. Aberrant recombination and the origin of Klinefelter syndrome. Hum Reprod Update. 2003;9:309-17.

25. Selice R, Di Mambro A, Garolla A, et al. Spermatogenesis in Klinefelter syndrome. J Endocrinol Invest. 2010;33:789-93.

26. Schlegel PN. Nonobstructive azoospermia: a revolutionary surgical approach and results. Semin Reprod Med. 2009;27:165-70.

27. Mehta A, Paduch DA. Klinefelter syndrome: an argument for early aggressive hormonal and fertility management. Fertl Steril. 2012;98(2):274-83.

28. Rommens JM, Iannuzzi MC, Kerem B, et al. Identification of the cystic fibrosis gene: chromosome walking and jumping. Science. 1989;245(4922):1059-65

29. Yu J, Chen Z, Ni Y, Li Z. CFTR mutations in men with congenital bilateral absence of the vas deferens (CBAVD): a systemic review and meta-analysis. Human Reprod. 2012;27(1):23-35.

30. Foresta C, Moro E, Ferlin A. Y chromosome microdeletions and alterations of spermatogenesis. Endocr Rev. 2001;22:226-39.

31. Massart A, Lissens W, Tournaye H, et al. Genetic causes of spermatogenic failure. Asian J Androl. 2012;14:40-48.

32. Sagnak L, Ersoy H, Ozok U, et al. The significance of Y chromosome microdeletion analysis in subfertile men with clinical variocele. Arch Med Sci. 2010;6(3):382-7.

33. Stahl PJ, Masson P, Mielnik A, et al. A decade of experience emphasizes that testing for Y microdeletions is essential in American men with azoospermia and severe oligozoospermia. Fertil Steril. 2010;;94(5):1753-6.

34. Sen S, Pasi AR, Dada R, et al. Y chromosome microdeletions in infertile men: prevalence, phenotypes and screening markers for the Indian population. J Assist Reprod Genet. 2013;30:413-22.

35. Sigman M, Jarow JP. Endocrine evaluation of infertile men. Urology. 1997;50: 659-64.

36. Kumar R. Medical management of non-obstructive azoospermia. Clinics. 2013;68(S1):75-9.

37. Potts JM, Pasqualotto FF, Nelson D, et al. Patient characteristics associated with vasectomy reversal. J Urol. 1999;161:1835-9.

38. Owen ER. Microsurgical vasovasostomy: a reliable vasectomy reversal. Aust NZJ Surg. 1977;47:305.

39. Silber SJ. Microscopic vasectomy reversal. Fertil Steril. 1977;28:1191.

40. Belker AM, Thomas AJ, Fuchs EF, et al. Results of 1,469 microsurgical vasectomy reversals by the Vasovasostomy Study Group. J Urol. 1991;145:505.

41. Ho Kl, Witte MN, Bird ET, et al. Fibrin glue assisted 3-suture vasovasostomy. J Urol. 2005;174(4Pt1):1360-63.

42. Fuchs EF, Burt RA. Vasectomy reversal performed 15 years or more after vasectomy: correlation of pregnancy outcome with partner age and with pregnancy results of in vitro fertilization with intracytoplasmic sperm injection. Fertil Steril. 2002;77:516-19.

43. Martin E, Carnett, JB, Levi JV, et al. The surgical treatment of sterility due to obstruction at the epididymis. Together with a study of the morphology of human spermatozoa. Univ Pa Med Bull. 1902;15:2-15.

44. Dubin L, Amelar RD. Magnified surgery for epididymovasostomy. Urology. 1984;23:525-8.

45. Schlegel PN, Goldstein M. Microsurgical vasoepididymostomy: refinements and results. J Urol. 1993;150:1165-8.

46. Schiff J, Chan P, Li PS, et al. Outcome and late failures compared in 4 techniques of micro- surgical vasoepididymostomy in 153 consecutive men. J Urol. 2005;174:651-5.

47. Smrkolj T, Virant-Klun I, Sinkovec J, et al. Epididymovasostomy as the first-line treatment of obstructive azoospermia in young couples with normal spermatogenesis. Reprod Biomed Online. 2010;20(5):594-601.

48. Lee HS, Seo JT. Advances in surgical treatment of male infertility. World J Mens Health. 2012;30(2):108-13.

49. Glina S, Vieira M. Prognostic factors for sperm retrieval in non-obstructive azoospermia. Clinics. 2013;68(S1):121-4.

CHAPTER
7
Surgical Management of Azoospermia

Rupin Shah

INTRODUCTION

With the introduction of microsurgical techniques for reconstructing cases of obstructive azoospermia (OA), and the use of intracytoplasmic sperm injection (ICSI) to directly achieve pregnancy in cases of both obstructive and nonobstructive azoospermia (NOA), a large proportion of azoospermic men can now father their own genetic child. The use of the correct surgical procedure is critical in obtaining the best outcome. Since the techniques of microsurgical reconstruction for OA and for sperm retrieval have been extensively described,[1-3] in this chapter, we focuses on the pros and cons of each procedure, and discuss the optimal approach to sperm retrieval. Operative procedures in azoospermia may be divided into:
- Reconstructive procedures (for OA)
    - *VEA*: Vasoepididymal anastomosis
    - *VVA*: Vasovasal anastomosis
    - *TURED*: Transurethral resection of ejaculatory duct
- Sperm retrieval procedures
    - Epididymal, percutaneous
        - *PESA*: Percutaneous epididymal sperm aspiration
    - Epididymal, open
        - *MESA*: Microsurgical epididymal sperm aspiration
    - Testicular, percutaneous
        - *TESA*: Testicular sperm aspiration
        - *NAB*: Needle aspiration biopsy
        - TruCut needle Biopsy
    - Testicular, open
        - Conventional open biopsy
        - *SST*: Single seminiferous tubule biopsies
        - *mdTESE*: Microdissection TESE

RECONSTRUCTIVE SURGERY

Vasoepididymal Anastomosis

VEA is performed for men with OA due to a block in the epididymis. Diagnosis is based on:

- Physical findings of a turgid epididymis and palpable normal vas
- Absence of inguinal or pelvic surgery (to rule out vas obstruction)
- Presence of fructose with normal semen volume (to rule out ejaculatory duct block)
- Normal spermatogenesis on testicular biopsy.

Several techniques have been described.[4] The older, conventional non-microsurgical VEA has been given up due to poor success rates. The currently preferred technique is a direct microsurgical anastomosis between a side-hole created in the epididymal ductule and the mucosa of the vas using 10-0 nylon. Patency rates average 50% and vary depending on the extent of epididymal damage and the etiology of the block. Half of those with a patent anastomosis will achieve a natural pregnancy.

ICSI vs VEA: Is a patient with epididymal obstruction better off with VEA or sperm aspiration and ICSI?

- Advantages of VEA
    - Allows a natural pregnancy
    - Second pregnancy possible without treatment
    - Corrects the primary problem
    - Saves the wife from unnecessary treatment
- Disadvantages of VEA
    - Needs special expertise in microsurgery
    - Can take 1 year for sperm to appear and even longer for pregnancy to occur
    - High failure rate if there is extensive epididymal damage
- Advantages of ICSI
    - Avoids need for a long, difficult surgical procedure
    - Much quicker results
    - Can be done when VEA has failed or has poor prognosis
    - More readily available than microsurgery
- Disadvantages of ICSI
    - Places burden of therapy on normal female partner, with attendant risks of hormonal stimulation and the IVF procedure
    - Needs to repeated for every pregnancy
    - More expensive than microsurgery
    - Not "natural"

Hence, VEA can be recommended when the couple is young and not in a hurry, or if they are insistent on a natural pregnancy, or if cost is a factor.

Intracytoplasmic sperm injection is recommended if the couple is ageing and there is no time to waste, or if the couple is in a hurry due to social reasons, or they are not interested in surgery, or if surgery has failed.

Vasovasal Anastomosis

The commonest reason for VVA is reversal of vasectomy.[5] In such cases, success depends on whether there is a secondary epididymal block due to back pressure from the vasectomy site. The longer the duration since vasectomy the greater is the likelihood of a secondary epididymal block.

If there is no epididymal block the technical success of microsurgical VVA[6] is over 90%. Hence, if the female partner is relatively young then VVA is more cost-effective than ICSI. If the female fertility is compromised then ART is a better option.

Transurethral Section of Ejaculatory Duct

Transurethral resection of ejaculatory duct is indicated when there is ejaculatory duct obstruction (EDO) with dilatation of the ejaculatory ducts (EjD). This is usually due to an intraprostatic cyst compressing the ejaculatory ducts. In such a case, the urologist can introduce a resectoscope and deroof the cyst by cutting the floor of the urethra near the veru. Occasionally, the block may be due to infection and the EjDs are individually dilated. Here surgery is more difficult since deroofing has to be more precise and there is a greater chance of restenosis.

However, EDO may also result from an infection (typically tuberculosis). In such cases, the EjDs are fibrosed and do not dilate; TUR is not possible, and sperm aspiration with ICSI is required.

This *important distinction between cystic and fibrous EDO* is made on the basis of a transrectal ultrasound (TRUS). In a man with azoospermia, low volume, absent fructose, and palpable vasa, if TRUS shows dilated seminal vesicles with intraprostatic dilatation of the EjD or an intraprostatic cyst then this is a cystic obstruction amenable to TURED. If TRUS shows nondilated EjDs and seminal vesicles this is indicative of a fibrous, nonoperable type of block.

SPERM RETRIEVAL PROCEDURES

Percutaneous Epididymal Sperm Aspiration

Sperm can be retrieved from the epididymis only in cases of OA. It is not indicated in men with NOA.

Percutaneous epididymal sperm aspiration is a simple procedure that involves percutaneous puncture of the epididymis with a fine needle and aspiration of epididymal fluid.[7] One may use a 24 gauge scalp vein connected to a syringe, or a tuberculin syringe with a 26 gauge needle (author's preference). The aspiration must be performed from the proximal epididymis (caput region) since in an obstructed system the distal sperm are old and degenerating and the best sperm are the most recent ones that are found in the caput.

Since the procedure is blind several punctures at different locations on the head may be required to get adequate numbers of motile sperm. Only motile epididymal sperm are used for ICSI since immotile epididymal sperm may be dead sperm.

Percutaneous epididymal sperm aspiration is easy and inexpensive, with no major complications, and can be repeated.[8] Hence, it has generally replaced the more complex MESA.

Microsurgical Epididymal Sperm Aspiration

Microsurgical epididymal sperm aspiration is the original technique described for sperm retrieval from the epididymis.[9] It involves open-surgical exposure of the epididymis and mobilization of a loop of epididymal ductule under magnification. The ductule in incised and the outpouring fluid is aspirated and checked for sperm. Once the flow stops the ductular opening is closed with microsutures. Multiple ductules can be opened at different locations so as to retrieve a large number of sperm.

While MESA allows for retrieval of a large number of sperm, adequate for many cycles of ICSI, it seems unnecessarily complex compared to PESA that can provide enough sperm in most cases.

Testicular Sperm Aspiration

Testicular sperm aspiration is like a fine-needle aspiration cytology of testis. A 24 gauge needle is attached to a syringe and suction is applied while making several passes through the testis. The aspirate is examined for sperm. FNAC of the testis has been used extensively both for diagnosis (to distinguish between OA and NOA) and for therapy, as a method of sperm retrieval. However, on both counts, it falls short.

Diagnostically, FNAC can be misleading because a few sperm may be seen in the aspirate even in cases of NOA with focal spermatogenesis. Thus, relying on FNAC to diagnose obstruction can lead to false explorations for corrective microsurgery.

Therapeutically, the opposite is also true for FNAC, it may fail to retrieve sperm in cases where there is only focal spermatogenesis. Several studies have compared sperm retrieval by FNAC versus tissue biopsy and have found fewer positive retrievals, and also fewer number of sperm retrieved.[10,11]

Hence, FNAC is better replaced by a needle biopsy that is equally non-invasive but more useful as described below.

Needle Aspiration Biopsy of the Testis

Needle aspiration biopsy differs from FNAC in that a larger bore scalp vein needle (18 gauge) is used. Suction is applied with a 10- or 20-mL syringe and the needle is passed in and out only in one direction, so that what is aspirated is not just fluid but a large chunk of testicular tissue containing many seminiferous tubules.[12] In fact, often the amount of tissue that is recovered by NAB may be more than traditionally removed by an open biopsy!

Diagnostically, NAB is equivalent to an open conventional biopsy because it provides tissue for histopathological examination, and when a four-quadrant NAB is performed it gives much more information than a single-open biopsy, while being less invasive or painful.

Therapeutically, NAB is far more efficient that FNAC in retrieving sperm since large amounts of tissue are available for processing. In fact, we find that doing a simple four-quadrant NAB in men with NOA is often sufficient to retrieve sperm and avoids the need for the more invasive open microsurgical sperm retrieval procedures.

TruCut Needle Biopsy of the Testis

Commercial needle biopsy systems may also be used to obtain testicular biopsy percutaneously,[13] but their cutting action makes them more traumatic than the NAB procedure with a scalp vein needle.

Conventional Open Biopsy

This is the traditional method of obtaining a testicular biopsy through a small incision in the skin and tunica. Performed correctly it is a simple and safe method of obtaining one or two diagnostic/therapeutic biopsies. However, in most cases the same tissue can usually be obtained by the NAB procedure that is less invasive. Hence, the author reserves diagnostic open biopsy for those cases where NAB fails due to fibrosis.

The conventional open biopsy has limited use for therapeutic sperm retrieval in men with testicular failure since, in these cases, often multiple biopsies are needed to find sperm. Each open biopsy can cause some degree of permanent testicular devascularization.[14,15] If sperm are retrieved within a couple of biopsies then no harm is done, but for a more extensive search the microsurgical techniques described below are more efficient and less harmful than multiple conventional open biopsies.

Single Seminiferous Tubule Biopsy Technique

This is an open microsurgical procedure that allows extensive sampling of the testis without the need for an incision in the tunica and with no risk of devascularization of testicular tissue.[16]

After exposure of the testis, an avascular area of the tunica is punctured with a fine needle. The opening is widened with the prong of a microforceps till a loop of seminiferous tubule pops out. This is grasped and pulled out and inspected under the operating microscope. If it appears promising then more tubule is extracted. If not, then another puncture is made a centimeter away and the procedure repeated. In this manner, the entire testicular surface can be mapped with 12–20 seminiferous tubule biopsies. The small punctures do not need any suturing and since no vessels are cut there is no damage to the testis. The SST technique is useful for sperm retrieval in men with testicular failure since it allows for extensive sampling while being less traumatic than mdTESE.

It may not be successful in very small or fibrotic testis in which no tissue protrudes through the puncture. In such cases, mdTESE is more useful.

Microdissection TESE

The testis is exposed and the tunica is incised along the circumference resulting in bivalving of the testis. The parenchyma is dissected and inspected under an operating microscope, looking for "fat" tubules that are more likely to contain sperm; these are biopsied. Thus, the entire testis is sampled with a large number of biopsies while removing only a small amount of tissue in total.[17,18]

Microdissection TESE offers the most thorough method for finding rare sperm in a case of testicular failure.[19] However, it is invasive and needs special training. There is risk of hematoma, infection and, rarely, atrophy if care is not taken to preserve vascularity.

Choice of Sperm Retrieval Technique

The technique to be used will depend on whether the man has OA or NOA.

In men in whom the distinction between OA and NOA is not clinically obvious, a diagnostic biopsy will be required. This should not only differentiate between OA and NOA, but also, in cases of NOA, identify whether focal spermatogenesis is present, and also obtain sperm for cryopreservation. Hence, for diagnosis, the single-open biopsy should be replaced by a four-quadrant NAB from both sides. One specimen would be sent for histopathology, while the rest go to the IVF laboratory for sperm retrieval, and cryopreservation if sperm are found. If no sperm are found in any of the eight biopsies then the patient can be counseled that the chances of finding sperm by mdTESE are < 10%.

For sperm retrieval in men with OA PESA is the technique of choice, offering a simple, painless method for retrieving a good number of motile sperm. When PESA is unsuccessful NAB or MESA can be done. In men with OA pregnancy rates are the same whether epididymal or testicular sperm are used.

In men with clinically obvious testicular failure, the author recommends a staged approach in one session. This is based on the finding that even in testicular failure, in the majority of cases where sperm are found these are in the first few biopsies,[20] but the occasional case will require a large number of biopsies. Start with four-quadrant NAB. If sperm are retrieved further invasive procedures can be avoided. If no sperm are retrieved then the testis is exposed and mapped by 18 SST biopsies. If still no sperm are found the procedure is extended into an mdTESE. If no sperm are found then the procedure is repeated on the opposite side.

With such a staged approach it will be possible to avoid the more aggressive open techniques in many men in whom sperm will be found by a simple (needle) biopsy.[21] At the same time, if sperm are not found by simpler methods the patient gets the benefit of the most effective method of sperm retrieval. The best chance is at the first attempt with higher transfer rates when fresh sperm are used;[22,23] hence, one should be prepared to offer all methods at the same session.

CONCLUSION

There have been many advances in the surgery for azoospermia, both in reconstructive procedures and in sperm retrieval techniques. Microsurgery plays an important role in optimizing results; choosing the right technique for sperm retrieval is very important.

REFERENCES

1. Marmar JL. Techniques for microsurgical reconstruction of obstructive azoospermia. Indian J Urol. 2011;27:86-91.
2. Donoso P, Tournaye H, Devroey P. Which is the best sperm retrieval technique for non-obstructive azoospermia. A systematic review? Hum Reprod Update. 2007;13:539-49.
3. Shah R. Surgical sperm retrieval: techniques and their indications. Indian J Urology. 2011;27:102-9.
4. Chan PT. The evolution and refinement of vasoepididymostomy techniques. Asian J Androl. 2013;15: 49-55.
5. Ramasamy R, Schlegel PN. Vasectomy and vasectomy reversal: an update. Indian J Urol. 2011;27:92-7.
6. Herrel L, Hsiao W. Microsurgical vasovasostomy. Asian J Androl. 2013;15:44-8.
7. Shrivastav P, Nadkarni P, Wensvoort S, et al. Percutaneous epididymal sperm aspiration for obstructive azoospermia. Hum Reprod. 1994;9:2058-61.

8. Rosenlund B, Westlander G, Wood M, et al. Sperm retrieval and fertilization in repeated percutaneous epididymal sperm aspiration. Hum Reprod. 1998; 13:2805-7.

9. Patrizio P, Silber S, Ord T, et al. Two births after microsurgical sperm aspiration in congenital absence of vas deferens. Lancet. 1988;2:1364.

10. Friedler S, Raziel A, Strassburger D, et al. Testicular sperm retrieval by percutaneous fine needle aspiration compared with testicular sperm extraction by open biopsy in men with NOA. Hum Reprod. 1997;12:1488-93.

11. Houwen J, Lundin K, Söderlund B, et al. Efficacy of percutaneous needle aspiration and open biopsy for sperm retrieval in men with non-obstructive azoospermia. Acta Obstet Gynecol Scand. 2008;87:1033-8.

12. Shah RS. Surgical and nonsurgical methods of sperm retrieval. In: Hansotia M, Desai S, Parihar M (Eds). Advanced Infertility Management. New Delhi: Jaypee Brothers; 2002. pp. 253-8.

13. Morey AF, Deshon GEJ, Rosanski TA, et al. Technique of biopty gun testis needle biopsy. Urology. 1993;42:325-6.

14. Schlegel PN, Su LM. Physiological consequences of testicular sperm extraction. Hum Reprod. 1997;12:1688-92.

15. Ron-El R, Strauss S, Friedler S, et al. Serial sonography and colour flow Doppler imaging following testicular and epididymal sperm extraction. Hum Reprod. 1998;13:3390-93.

16. Shah RS. Operative sperm retrieval for ART. In: Goenka ML, Goenka D (Eds). Recent Advances in Infertility Management. Guwahati: Goenka; 2001. pp. 179-83.

17. Schlegel PN, Li PS. Microdissection TESE: sperm retrieval in non-obstructive azoospermia. Hum Reprod Update. 1998;4:439.

18. Schlegel PN. Testicular sperm extraction: microdissection improves sperm yield with minimal tissue excision. Hum Reprod. 1999;14:131-5.

19. Schlegel PN. Nonobstructive azoospermia: a revolutionary surgical approach and results. Semin Reprod Med. 2009;27:165-70.

20. Altay S, Hekimgil M, Cikili N, et al. Histopathological mapping of open testicular biopsies in patients with unobstructed azoospermia. Br J Urol Int. 2001;87:834-7.

21. Colpi GM, Colpi EM, Piediferro G, et al. Microsurgical TESE versus conventional TESE for ICSI in non-obstructive azoospermia: a randomized controlled study. Reprod Biomed Online. 2009;18:315-9.

22. Verheyen G, Vernaeve V, Van Landuyt L, et al. Should diagnostic testicular sperm retrieval followed by cryopreservation for later ICSI be the procedure of choice for all patients with non-obstructive azoospermia? Hum Reprod. 2004;19:2822-30.

23. Craft I, Tsirigotis M. Simplified recovery, preparation and cryopreservation of testicular sperm. Hum Reprod. 1995;10:1623-27.

Index

Page numbers followed by *f* refer to figure and *t* refer to table.